theclinics.com

CRITICAL CARE CLINICS

Pharmacotherapy

GUEST EDITORS
Steven J. Martin, PharmD, BCPS, FCCP, FCCM
Joseph F. Dasta, MSc, FCCM

CONSULTING EDITORS
Richard W. Carlson, MD, PhD
Michael A. Geheb, MD

April 2006 • Volume 22 • Number 2

SAUNDERS
An Imprint of Elsevier, Inc.
PHILADELPHIA LONDON TORONTO MONTREAL SYDNEY TOKYO

W.B. SAUNDERS COMPANY
A Division of Elsevier Inc.

Elsevier Inc. • 1600 John F. Kennedy Blvd., Suite 1800 • Philadelphia, Pennsylvania 19103-2899

http://www.theclinics.com

CRITICAL CARE CLINICS **Volume 22, Number 2**
April 2006 **ISSN 0749-0704**
Editor: Maria Lorusso **ISBN 1-4160-3516-8**

Reprints. For copies of 100 or more, of articles in this publication, please contact the Commercial Reprints Department, Elsevier Inc., 360 Park Avenue South, New York, New York 10010-1710. Phone: (212) 633-3813; Fax: (212) 462-1935; E-mail: reprints@elsevier.com

Critical Care Clinics (ISSN 0749-0704) is published quarterly by W.B. Saunders Company. Corporate and editorial offices: Elsevier Inc., 1600 John F. Kennedy Blvd., Philadelphia, PA 19103-2899. Accounting and circulation offices: 6277 Sea Harbor Drive, Orlando, FL 32887-4800. Periodicals postage paid at Orlando, FL 32862, and additional mailing offices. Subscription prices are $170.00 per year for US individuals, $280.00 per year for US institution, $85.00 per year for US students and residents, $210.00 per year for Canadian individuals, $340.00 per year for Canadian institutions, $230.00 per year for international individuals, $340.00 per year for international institutions and $115.00 per year for Canadian and foreign students/residents. To receive student/resident rate, orders must be accompanied by name of affiliated institution, date of term, and the *signature* of program/residency coordinator on institution letterhead. Orders will be billed at individual rate until proof of status is received. Foreign air speed delivery is included in all *Clinics* subscription prices. All prices are subject to change without notice. POSTMASTER: Send address changes to *Critical Care Clinics,* W.B. Saunders Company, Periodicals Fulfillment, Orlando, FL 32887-4800. **Customer Service: 1-800-654-2452 (US). From outside of the US, call 1-407-345-1000. E-mail: hhspcs@harcourt.com**

Critical Care Clinics is also published in Spanish by Editorial Inter-Medica, Junin 917, 1er A, 1113, Buenos Aires, Argentina.

Critical Care Clinics is covered in *Index Medicus, EMBASE/Excerpta Medica, Current Concepts/Clinical Medicine, ISI/BIOMED,* and *Chemical Abstracts.*

Printed in the United States of America.

CONSULTING EDITORS

RICHARD W. CARLSON, MD, PhD, Chairman, Department of Internal Medicine, Marcopia Medical Center; and Professor, Department of Medicine, Mayo Graduate School of Medicine, Phoenix, Arizona

MICHAEL A. GEHEB, MD, Professor, Department of Medicine, and Vice President, Clinical Programs, Oregon Health & Sciences University, Portland, Oregon

GUEST EDITORS

STEVEN J. MARTIN, PharmD, BCPS, FCCP, FCCM, The University of Toledo, Toledo, Ohio

JOSEPH F. DASTA, MSc, FCCM, Professor, College of Pharmacy, The Ohio State University, Columbus, Ohio

CONTRIBUTORS

BRADLEY A. BOUCHER, PharmD, BCPS, FCCP, FCCM, Professor of Pharmacy, Department of Pharmacy; Associate Professor of Neurosurgery, Department of Neurosurgery, University of Tennessee Health Science Center, Memphis, Tennessee

JOSEPH F. DASTA, MSc, FCCM, Professor, College of Pharmacy, The Ohio State University, Columbus, Ohio

REED E. DREWS, MD, Associate Professor, Department of Medicine, Division of Hematology-Oncology; Director, Hematology-Oncology Training Program, Beth Israel Deaconess Medical Center, Harvard Medical School, Boston, Massachusetts

E. WESLEY ELY, MD, MPH, Department of Medicine, Center for Health Services Research, and Division of Allergy/Pulmonary/Critical Care Medicine, Vanderbilt University School of Medicine, Nashville, Tennessee; and the Center for Health Services Research and the Veterans Administration Tennessee Valley Geriatric Research, Education, and Clinical Center, Tennessee

DAVID FELDMAN, MD, PhD, Director of Heart Failure and Cardiac Transplantation, Departments of Medicine/Cardiology & Physiology and Cell Biology, The Ohio State University, Columbus, Ohio

DOUGLAS N. FISH, PharmD, FCCM, Associate Professor and Vice Chair, Department of Clinical Pharmacy, School of Pharmacy, University of Colorado Health Sciences Center; and Clinical Specialist, Critical Care/Infectious Diseases, Department of Pharmacy, University of Colorado Hospital, Denver, Colorado

JUDITH JACOBI, PharmD, FCCM, FCCP, BCPS, Critical Care Pharmacist, Pharmacy Department, Methodist Hospital/Clarian Health Partners, Indianapolis, Indiana

SANDRA KANE-GILL, PharmD, MSc, Assistant Professor, School of Pharmacy, University of Pittsburgh, Pittsburgh, Pennsylvania

XI LIU-DERYKE, PharmD, Neuroscience Research Fellow, Department of Pharmacy Practice, Eugene Applebaum College of Pharmacy and Health Sciences, Wayne State University, Detroit, Michigan

HENRY J. MANN, PharmD, Professor, Department of Experimental and Clinical Pharmacology, College of Pharmacy; Director, Center for Excellence in Critical Care, University of Minnesota, Minneapolis, Minnesota

ALEXANDRE MEBAZAA, MD, PhD, Professor and Director, Department of Anesthesiology and Critical Care Medicine, Hopitale Laribiosiere, Paris, France

BRUCE A. MUELLER, PharmD, FCCP, Professor and Chair, Department of Clinical Sciences, University of Michigan College of Pharmacy, Ann Arbor, Michigan

TIEN M.H. NG, PharmD, Assistant Professor, Department of Pharmacy, University of Southern California, Los Angeles, California

MARTIN J. OHLINGER, PharmD, Assistant Professor, Department of Pharmacy Practice, University of Toledo College of Pharmacy; and Clinical Pharmacy Specialist, Medical University of Ohio University Medical Center, Toledo, Ohio

PRATIK PANDHARIPANDE, MD, MSCI, Division of Critical Care, Department of Anesthesiology, Vanderbilt University School of Medicine, Nashville, Tennessee

DENISE H. RHONEY, PharmD, FCCP, Associate Professor, Department of Pharmacy Practice, Eugene Applebaum College of Pharmacy and Health Sciences, Wayne State University, Detroit, Michigan

AMARDEEP K. SINGH, MD, Department of Internal Medicine, University of Southern California, Los Angeles, California

JOSEPH M. SWANSON, PharmD, BCPS, Critical Care Pharmacy Fellow, Department of Pharmacy, University of Tennessee Health Science Center, Memphis, Tennessee

STEPHANIE S. TABER, PharmD, Clinical Assistant Professor, Department of Clinical Sciences, University of Michigan College of Pharmacy, Ann Arbor, Michigan

ERIK R. VANDENDRIES, MD, PhD, Research Fellow, Division of Hemostasis/Thrombosis, Beth Israel Deaconess Medical Center, Boston; and Associate Medical Director, PAREXEL International, Waltham, Massachusetts

JEAN-LOUIS VINCENT, MD, PhD, Service des Soins Intensifs, Hôpital Universitaire Erasme, Brussels, Belgium

ROBERT J. WEBER, MSc, FASHP, Associate Professor, School of Pharmacy; Chairman, Department of Pharmacy and Therapeutics, University of Pittsburgh, Pittsburgh; and Executive Director of Pharmacy, University of Pittsburgh Medical Center, Pittsburgh, Pennsylvania

G. CHRISTOPHER WOOD, PharmD, BCPS, Associate Professor of Pharmacy, Department of Pharmacy, University of Tennessee Health Science Center, Memphis, Tennessee

CONTENTS

FORTHCOMING ISSUES

July 2006

International Perspectives in Critical Care Medicine
Jose Besso, MD, *Guest Editor*

October 2006

Neurologic Critical Care
Romergryko G. Geocadin, MD, and
Robert D. Stevens, MD, *Guest Editors*

January 2007

Early Mobility and ICU Outcome
Peter E. Morris, MD, *Guest Editor*

RECENT ISSUES

January 2006

Endocrinology of Critical Illness
Greet Van den Berghe, MD, PhD, *Guest Editor*

October 2005

Terrorism and Critical Care: Chemical, Biologic, Radiologic, and Nuclear Weapons
Jerris R. Hedges, MD, MS, and
Robert G. Hendrickson, MD, *Guest Editors*

July 2005

Hematology Issues in Critical Illness
Per Thorborg, MD, PhD, and
Lynn K. Boshkov, MD, *Guest Editors*

ELSEVIER
SAUNDERS

Crit Care Clin 22 (2006) xi–xii

CRITICAL
CARE
CLINICS

Preface

Pharmacotherapy

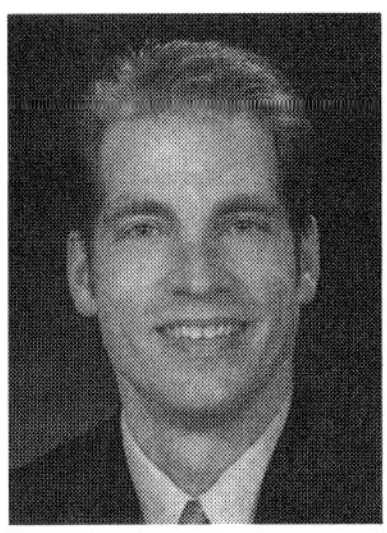
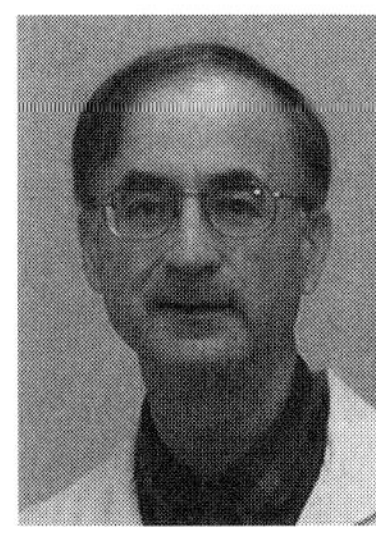

Steven J. Martin, PharmD, BCPS, FCCP, FCCM   Joseph F. Dasta, MSc, FCCM
Guest Editors

Critical care medicine is an evolving science, and drug use, or pharmacotherapy, plays an integral role in optimizing outcomes for our patients. As knowledge has expanded to better understand the complex mechanisms of the pathophysiology common to the ICU patient, so too has the understanding of the mechanisms, pharmacokinetics, pharmacodynamics, and interactions of drugs used in this setting. Drug therapy is the primary method of treating diseases of critical illness, including heart disease, endocrine disorders, neurologic disorders, and infectious disease, among others. However, the disposition of medications in the ICU patient is altered by critical illness, and this process changes over time. Hence, dosing drugs used in the ICU is a complex process. All too often, the therapies themselves become a cause of the disease, resulting from either under- or overdosing.

It is these principles that this edition of the *Critical Care Clinics* addresses. Evidence-based reviews and practical issues surrounding the therapy of major diseases affecting the critically ill are provided, along with a section on pharmacokinetic changes of critical illness and drug-induced disease. The authors of this edition are outstanding clinicians and scientists who have contributed significantly to the literature in the area of pharmacotherapy. Critical care medicine is at a pivotal point in the history of the discipline. Drug therapy today is complex and interconnected. Novel chemicals that transcend the traditional drug–receptor

doi:10.1016/j.ccc.2006.03.001

interaction have made surgical precision of drug, dose, route, and frequency the nexus to restoration of health. Pharmacotherapy offers the greatest potential for future leaps in improvement, not only in the survival from critical illness, but also in the mitigation of discomfort and the palliation of suffering in both the short and long term for patients.

Steven J. Martin, PharmD, BCPS, FCCP, FCCM
The University of Toldeo
College of Pharmacy
2801 West Bancroft Street
Toledo, OH 43606, USA
E-mail address: steven.martin@utoledo.edu

Joseph F. Dasta, MSc, FCCM
The Ohio Sate University
College of Pharmacy
500 West 12th Avenue
Columbus, OH 43210-1291, USA
E-mail address: dasta.1@osu.edu

ELSEVIER
SAUNDERS

Crit Care Clin 22 (2006) 187–197

CRITICAL
CARE
CLINICS

Vasopressin in Hypotensive and Shock States

Jean-Louis Vincent, MD, PhD

Service des Soins Intensifs, Hôpital Universitaire Erasme, Route de Lennik 808, Brussels B-1070, Belgium

Vasopressin is a relatively recent member of the therapeutic armamentarium for shock, although it has been well conserved through evolution and its ancestral gene probably dates back more than 700 million years. The characterization by Oliver and Schaefer [1] more than 100 years ago of the vasopressor effects of a substance produced by the neurohypophysis led, some 50 years later, to the description of the structure of vasopressin by du Vigneaud, for which, along with his work on oxytocin, he won the Nobel Prize for chemistry. For many years termed *antidiuretic hormone* because of its effects on the distal tubule of the kidney, it is only relatively recently that interest has been rekindled in the vasopressor effects of vasopressin and its possible role in patients with shock.

Physiologic role of vasopressin

Vasopressin is synthesized by the magnocellular neurons of the hypothalamus and stored in the posterior lobe of the pituitary gland. Vasopressin is involved in the maintenance of blood osmolality and volume, by its effects on the kidneys, and in the control of blood pressure, by its constrictor effects on vascular smooth muscle [2]. It also has a broad range of other functions, including effects on body temperature, on insulin release [3], on corticotropin release [4], on memory [5], and on social behavior [6]. It achieves these effects by interaction with G-protein–coupled vasopressin-specific receptors, of which there are at least three main types: V1, V2, and VS (or V1b) [2,7,8]. V1 receptors are located on vascular smooth muscle cells and mediate vasopressin's effects on arterial blood pressure via a variety of signaling pathways, including calcium influx and

E-mail address: jlvincen@ulb.ac.be

doi:10.1016/j.ccc.2006.02.012 ***criticalcare.theclinics.com***

activation of phospholipases [8]. In the pulmonary circulation, vasopressin activation of V1 receptors causes release of nitric oxide (NO), with resultant vasodilatation and decreased pulmonary vascular resistance [9]. V1 receptors are also found in the kidney, where vasopressin causes reduced blood flow to the inner medulla without influencing outer medullary flow [10]. V2 receptors are found on the distal convoluted tubule and medullary collecting ducts of the kidney and mediate the antidiuretic effects of vasopressin, primarily signaling via cyclic adenosine monophosphate (cAMP). V3 receptors are found in the anterior hypophysis, where they are involved in stimulating corticotropin release. Vasopressin can also bind to oxytocin receptors, which are present in high density on vascular endothelium, where it increases intracellular calcium, stimulating release of NO and causing vasodilation. The effects of vasopressin on P2 purinoreceptors [11] may cause coronary vasoconstriction.

Vasopressin is normally released in response to decreased blood pressure, reduced blood volume, or increased plasma osmolality, with secretion being regulated by various mechanisms, including hypothalamic osmoreceptors, left atrial stretch receptors, and arterial baroreceptors (Fig. 1). Pain, nausea, hypoxia, and pharyngeal stimuli as well as endogenous and exogenous chemicals, such as norepinephrine and acetylcholine, can also increase the release of vasopressin [12]. Plasma vasopressin concentrations seem to be more sensitive to changes in plasma osmolality than to changes in blood pressure or volume [2], and in

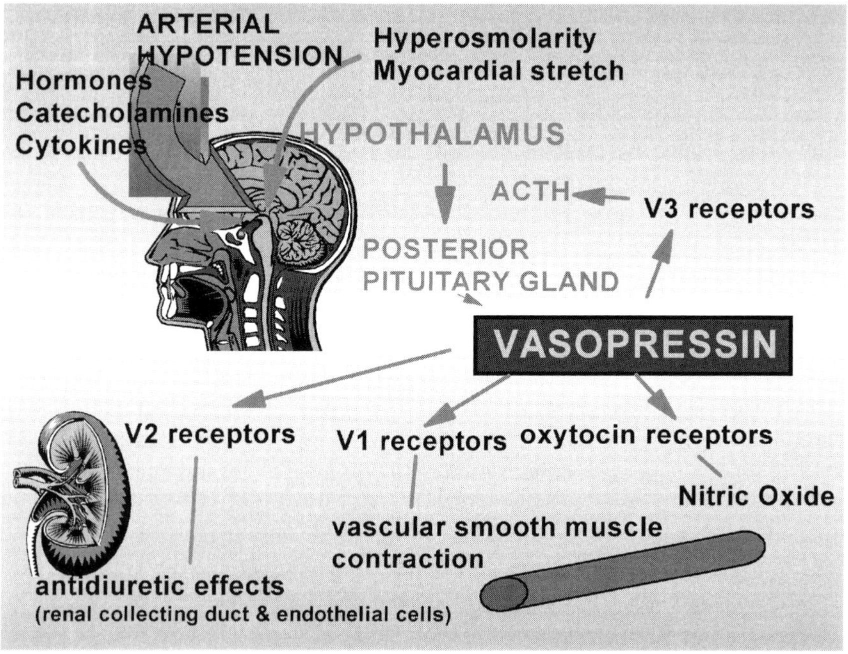

Fig. 1. Schematic representation of key factors involved in regulation and secretion of endogenous vasopressin.

physiologic conditions, vasopressin's main role is the regulation of water balance [13]. It does not seem to play a major role in the vascular regulation of blood pressure, and, indeed, the syndrome of inappropriate antidiuretic hormone secretion, where endogenous vasopressin concentrations are abnormally high, is not associated with hypertension. The normal plasma vasopressin concentration in a hemodynamically stable subject is 2.2 to 4.0 pg/mL for a serum osmolality of less than 285 mOsm/kg [14].

Vasopressin in shock

In shock, hypotension stimulates vasopressin release, and high concentrations can be reached rapidly after the onset of hypotension whether attributable to cardiac arrest, hemorrhage, epidural anesthesia, septic shock, or even exercise [13]. The high concentrations of vasopressin cause vasoconstriction by several mechanisms, including activation of V1 receptors, modulation of ATP-sensitive K+ channels, modulation of NO, and potentiation of adrenergic and other vasoconstrictor agents, including norepinephrine and angiotensin II [15], helping to restore and maintain blood pressure. Vasopressin's seemingly paradoxic vasodilatory effect depends on which vascular bed is being studied and the dose of and duration of exposure to vasopressin. Further study is needed to understand the relation between vasopressin's vasodilatory and vasoconstrictive actions.

Clinical studies of vasopressin in shock

The effects of vasopressin have been studied in various groups of patients with vasodilatory shock [16–23]. Argenziano and colleagues [16] randomized 10 patients with vasodilatory shock requiring catecholamine vasopressors after placement of a left ventricular assist device to vasopressin at a rate of 0.1 U/min or to saline placebo. Patients who received vasopressin increased their mean arterial pressure (57 $\pm$ 4 to 84 $\pm$ 2 mm Hg; $P<.001$) and systemic vascular resistance (813 $\pm$ 113 to 1188 $\pm$ 87 dyne-s/cm^5; $P<.001$) and had reduced norepinephrine requirements. Interestingly, all subjects responded to vasopressin administration regardless of their vasopressin concentrations before randomization. Morales and coworkers [18] also reported, in a retrospective chart review of 50 patients with vasodilatory shock after placement of a left ventricular assist device, that vasopressin administration (0.09 $\pm$ 0.05 U/min) increased mean arterial pressure (58 $\pm$ 13 to 75 $\pm$ 14 mm Hg; $P<.001$) and reduced norepinephrine requirements. Argenziano and colleagues [17] reported similar results in a small group of patients with vasodilatory shock after cardiac transplantation. In patients with severe congestive heart failure and milrinone-induced hypotension, vasopressin (0.03–0.07 U/min) increased systolic arterial pressure (from 90 $\pm$ 3 to 127 $\pm$ 2 mm Hg; $P<.01$) and allowed for a decrease in the dosage and the frequency of administration of norepinephrine [19]. Interestingly, Morales and coworkers [24] investigated whether vasopressin given prophylactically (0.03 U/min) before cardiopulmonary bypass would diminish postbypass hypotension and catecholamine use by avoiding vasopressin deficiency. The authors reported that patients who received vasopressin before bypass had a lower peak norepinephrine dose than those who received placebo (4.6 ± 2.5 versus 7.3 ± 3.5 μg/min; $P = .03$), a shorter duration of catecholamines (5 ± 6 versus 11 ± 7 hours; $P = .03$), and a shorter intensive care unit (ICU) length of stay (1.2 ± 0.4 versus 2.1 ± 1.4 days; $P = .03$). Early administration of low-dose vasopressin would therefore seem to be beneficial in vasodilatory shock, although no large studies have been published that demonstrate an effect on outcome.

Vasopressin in septic shock

In patients with septic shock, as in other forms of shock, vasopressin concentrations rise sharply, but they then decrease to concentrations unexpectedly low for the level of hypotension [25,26]. Landry and coworkers [26] reported that in 19 patients with septic shock, vasopressin concentrations were 3.1 ± 0.4 pg/mL compared with the concentrations of 22.7 ± 2.2 pg/mL seen in 12 patients with cardiogenic shock and hypotension of similar duration.

The mechanism underlying these reduced vasopressin concentrations is unclear. Possible mechanisms include depletion of vasopressin stores, inhibition of vasopressin release, alterations of the autonomic nervous system, and increased vasopressin degradation. The administration of vasopressin at a rate of 0.01 U/min to two septic shock patients increased plasma vasopressin concentrations to 27 and 34 pg/mL, respectively [26], and others have also reported increased plasma concentrations after vasopressin administration [27], suggesting that increased catabolism of vasopressin is not responsible for the reduced concentrations. Impaired baroreflex-mediated vasopressin secretion may be implicated, but vasopressin does not seem to induce bradycardia when given in septic shock [26], although bradycardia is seen when vasopressin is used in physiologic conditions [28]. In three patients, Sharshar and colleagues [29] reported depleted vasopressin stores in the neurohypophysis as assessed by MRI. There was no detectable vasopressinase activity, suggesting that increased elimination of vasopressin is unlikely to be responsible for the reduced concentrations. Hence, reduced vasopressin production would seem to be at least partly responsible for the low vasopressin response seen in patients with septic shock [30].

Clinical studies of vasopressin in septic shock

After the findings of Landry and coworkers [26], vasopressin has been studied as a potential vasopressor agent in patients with septic shock [14,20,26,31–35]. Although no study has yet shown any positive effect on outcome with vasopressin use, hemodynamic parameters and urine output seem to improve. The earliest studies were case series by Landry and coworkers [14,26]. In five patients with septic shock, Landry and coworkers [14] noted that vasopressin infusion (0.01–0.05 U/min) increased arterial pressure in all patients and restored urine output in three of the five patients. In 10 patients with septic shock who were receiving catecholamines, vasopressin administration at a rate of 0.04 U/min increased systolic arterial pressure from 92 to 146 mm Hg ($P < .001$) because of peripheral vasoconstriction (systemic vascular resistance increased from 644 to 1187 dyne.s/cm^5; $P < .001$) [26]. The same authors [26] also noted that in six patients with septic shock who were receiving vasopressin as the sole vasopressor, withdrawal of vasopressin resulted in hypotension. Vasopressin administered at a dose of 0.01 U/min, which resulted in a plasma concentration expected for the level of hypotension, increased systolic pressure from 83 to 115 mm Hg ($P < .01$). In a small, randomized, controlled trial of 10 trauma patients with septic shock, Malay and colleagues [31] reported that vasopressin (0.04 U/min) increased arterial pressure and systemic vascular resistance, whereas placebo (saline) had no effect on these parameters. Patel and coworkers [34] randomized patients with septic shock refractory to high-dose vasopressor agents to an infusion of vasopressin (0.01–0.08 U/min) or norepinephrine (2–16 μg/min). Vasopressin infusion spared conventional vasopressor use and improved creatinine clearance compared with norepinephrine.

Other effects of vasopressin infusion

Hepatosplanchnic perfusion

In all the reported studies [14,20,26,31–35], low-dose vasopressin infusion has been shown to improve systemic blood pressure without significant adverse effects on cardiac or pulmonary hemodynamics. Its strong vasoconstrictive properties raise concern about possible hypoperfusion to various organs, however, including the splanchnic region. The data regarding vasopressin's effects on the hepatosplanchnic circulation are conflicting. Martikainen and colleagues [36] reported impaired splanchnic perfusion during vasopressin infusion in endotoxic pigs. Also in endotoxic pigs, Asfar and coworkers [37] reported that terlipressin, a lysine vasopressin analogue, increased hepatic artery flow and attenuated the hepatosplanchnic venous acidosis. Malay and colleagues [38] noted that low-dose vasopressin did not impair blood flow to the renal or mesenteric beds in pigs with endotoxic shock but that higher doses of vasopressin reduced mesenteric and renal blood flow. Most recently, Knotzer and coworkers [39] reported no detrimental effects of vasopressin in jejunal mucosal oxygenation after vasopressin infusion in pigs with acute endotoxic shock.

In a sheep model of peritonitis-induced septic shock, we studied the effects of vasopressin (0.02 U/min), norepinephrine (0.5–5 μg/kg/min titrated to maintain mean arterial pressure between 75 and 85 mm Hg), or vasopressin (0.01 U/min) plus norepinephrine (0.5–5 μg/kg/min titrated to maintain mean arterial pressure between 75 and 85 mm Hg) [40]. Although mean arterial pressure was well

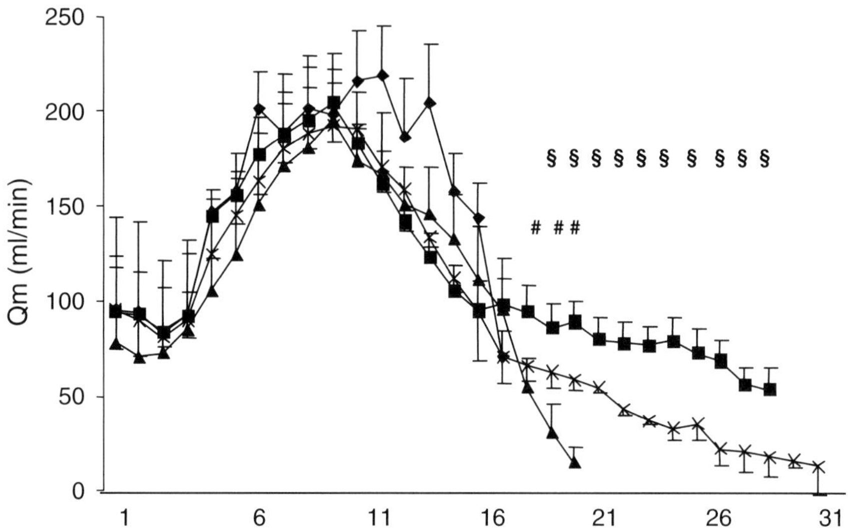

Fig. 2. Changes in mesenteric blood flow (Qm) for the four groups of sheep: control (CL, ◆), vasopressin (VP, ■), norepinephrine (NE, ▲), and VP+NE (X). #$p<0.05$ NE vs VP; $$p<0.05$ VPNE vs VP. (*Modified from* Sun Q, Dimopoulos G, Nguyen DN, et al. Low-dose vasopressin in the treatment of septic shock in sheep. Am J Respir Crit Care Med 2003;168(4):483; with permission.)

maintained in all three groups, superior mesenteric arterial blood flow was significantly higher in the vasopressin group than in the other groups (Fig. 2). The survival time was longer in sheep given vasopressin than in those that did not receive it (Fig. 3).

Clinical studies have also reported conflicting reports of the effects of vasopressin on hepatosplanchnic perfusion. In 11 patients with septic shock receiv-

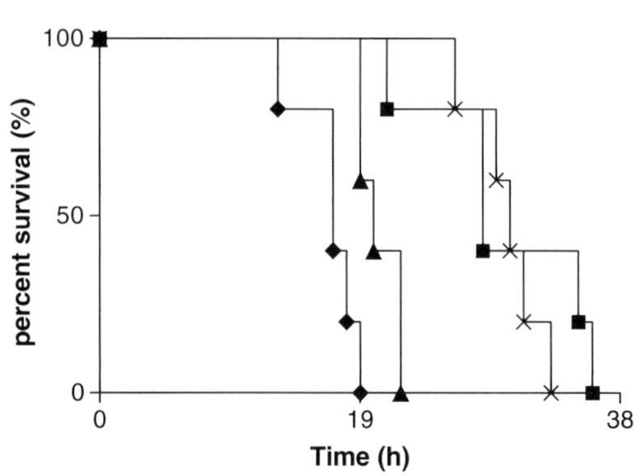

Fig. 3. Kaplan-Meier survival curves for the four groups of sheep: control (CL, ◆), vasopressin (VP, ■), norepinephrine (NE, ▲), and VP + NE (×). $P<.05$, CL versus VP, NE, or VP + NE. (*From* Sun Q, Dimopoulos G, Nguyen DN, et al. Low-dose vasopressin in the treatment of septic shock in sheep. Am J Respir Crit Care Med 2003;168(4):484; with permission.)

ing norepinephrine infusion, vasopressin infusion (0.04 U/min) resulted in an increase in the median gastric partial pressure of carbon dioxide ($PgCO_2$) gap from 5 to 19 mm Hg ($P = .022$) [41]. In 12 patients with septic shock, Klinzing and colleagues [42] reported that replacement of norepinephrine infusion with vasopressin (0.06–1.8 IU/min) resulted in an increase in the $PgCO_2$ gap from 17.5 $\pm$ 26.6 to 36.5 $\pm$ 26.6 mm Hg ($P < .01$). Morelli and coworkers [43] reported that terlipressin reduced the $PgCO_2$ gap in 15 patients with norepinephrine-treated septic shock, however. Dunser and colleagues [44] found that gastrointestinal perfusion as assessed by gastric tonometry was better preserved in patients treated with vasopressin than in those who received norepinephrine or norepinephrine with vasopressin.

Renal blood flow

Vasopressin has complex effects on the kidney. Although it may reduce urine output to maintain blood volume, it can also have a diuretic effect in septic shock, believed to be, at least in part, attributable to greater vasoconstriction of the efferent arteriole than the afferent arteriole [45]. In the study by Sun and colleagues [40] in sheep with peritonitis-induced septic shock, vasopressin infusion (with or without norepinephrine) resulted in higher urine output than in sheep that did not receive vasopressin. Most, although not all [46], clinical studies have reported that vasopressin (and terlipressin) can improve urine output [32–34,43].

Adverse effects

Vasopressin is a potent vasoconstrictor of skin vessels, and extravasation of vasopressin can cause severe local skin necrosis [47]. Vasopressin infusion is also associated with ischemic skin lesions at sites other than the infusion site [48]. Concerns have also been raised about possible alterations in liver function and decreased platelet counts [20,49,50], but the clinical significance of these effects is unclear.

How should we use vasopressin?

Clinical reports and experimental studies certainly support the beneficial effects of low-dose vasopressin infusions in vasodilatory shock. Nevertheless, is an increase in arterial pressure, and perhaps in urine output, sufficient to support the use of vasopressin in all patients with septic shock? Although recent animal studies have suggested improved outcomes in animals treated with vasopressin [40], no clinical study has yet demonstrated reduced mortality in patients treated with vasopressin. The results of the recently completed vasopressin versus norepinephrine in septic shock (VASST) study comparing low-dose vasopressin with norepinephrine are eagerly awaited and should shed some light on the role of vasopressin in septic shock. Nevertheless, we are currently left with several unanswered questions. First, should vasopressin be considered as a vasopressor therapy (after all, it has vasopressor effects), as endocrine support (after all, it is a hormone), or both [30]? In hypotensive septic shock, the catecholamine α_1-adrenergic receptors may be desensitized or downregulated to standard catecholamine vasopressors, limiting their vasopressor activity [51]. Because vasopressin binds to its own V1 vascular receptor, it can still act to restore vascular tone even if the catecholamine α_1-adrenergic receptors are downregulated. Several clinical studies have reported that catecholamine requirements are reduced during vasopressin administration [14,20,31,32,34]. Although it certainly has vasopressor effects, there is no suggestion that vasopressin should be used like conventional agents and titrated to arterial pressure. Rather, if given, it should be used at low fixed dosages. Current guidelines on the management of septic shock suggest that vasopressin use may be considered in patients with refractory septic shock despite adequate fluid resuscitation and high-dose conventional vasopressors [52]. So, if we are using vasopressin more as endocrinologic support, should we only be giving it to patients with low vasopressin concentrations? Sharshar and colleagues [25] suggested that relative vasopressin deficiency occurred in only one third of late septic shock patients, and Jochberger and coworkers [53] reported that it was present in only 22% of their patients with septic shock 24 hours after ICU admission. In addition, the effects of vasopressin on arterial pressure seem to occur regardless of the endogenous plasma vasopressin concentration [16,54]. These observations suggest that vasopressin therapy may be beneficial in all patients with septic shock rather than only in those with low vasopressin concentrations [55].

Interestingly, Lin and colleagues [56] recently proposed that a low vasopressin/norepinephrine ratio could predict the development of septic shock in emergency department patients with sepsis or severe sepsis, suggesting that the changes in vasopressin occur before shock develops. In their patients, the plasma vasopressin concentration at baseline was significantly lower for those who finally developed septic shock (septic shock group, 3.6 ± 2.5 pg/mL; 95% confidence interval [CI], 3.0–4.2 pg/mL; severe sepsis group, 21.8 ± 4.1 pg/mL, 95% CI, 20.7–22.9 pg/mL; sepsis group, 10.6 ± 6.5 pg/mL, 95% CI, 8.8–12.4 pg/mL; $P < .001$). These findings would suggest that vasopressin should perhaps be given early rather than as a last resort in patients with intractable shock.

Summary

The results of experimental and clinical studies have so far been encouraging; however, clearly, many questions remain unanswered. Before we can recommend vasopressin for routine clinical use in vasodilatory shock, and particularly septic shock, we must await the results of currently ongoing and recently completed randomized clinical trials to ensure that vasopressin does indeed have beneficial effects on organ function and outcome.

References

[1] Oliver G, Schaefer EA. On the physiological action of extract of pituitary body and certain other glandular organs. J Physiol 1895;18:277–9.

[2] Mutlu GM, Factor P. Role of vasopressin in the management of septic shock. Intensive Care Med 2004;30(7):1276–91.

[3] Oshikawa S, Tanoue A, Koshimizu TA, et al. Vasopressin stimulates insulin release from islet cells through V1b receptors: a combined pharmacological/knockout approach. Mol Pharmacol 2004;65(3):623–9.

[4] Tanoue A, Ito S, Honda K, et al. The vasopressin V1b receptor critically regulates hypothalamic-pituitary-adrenal axis activity under both stress and resting conditions. J Clin Invest 2004; 113(2):302–9.

[5] Weingartner H, Gold P, Ballenger JC, et al. Effects of vasopressin on human memory functions. Science 1981;211(4482):601–3.

[6] Bielsky IF, Hu SB, Ren X, et al. The V1a vasopressin receptor is necessary and sufficient for normal social recognition: a gene replacement study. Neuron 2005;47(4):503–13.

[7] Thibonnier M, Coles P, Thibonnier A, et al. Molecular pharmacology and modeling of vasopressin receptors. Prog Brain Res 2002;139:179–96.

[8] Holmes CL, Landry DW, Granton JT. Science review: vasopressin and the cardiovascular system: part 1—receptor physiology. Crit Care 2003;7(6):427–34.

[9] Evora PR, Pearson PJ, Schaff HV. Arginine vasopressin induces endothelium-dependent vasodilatation of the pulmonary artery. V1-receptor-mediated production of nitric oxide. Chest 1993;103(4):1241–5.

[10] Bankir L. Antidiuretic action of vasopressin: quantitative aspects and interaction between V1a and V2 receptor-mediated effects. Cardiovasc Res 2001;51(3):372–90.

[11] Zenteno-Savin T, Sada-Ovalle I, Ceballos G, et al. Effects of arginine vasopressin in the heart are mediated by specific intravascular endothelial receptors. Eur J Pharmacol 2000;410(1):15–23.

[12] Holmes CL, Patel BM, Russell JA, et al. Physiology of vasopressin relevant to management of septic shock. Chest 2001;120(3):989–1002.

[13] Forrest P. Vasopressin and shock. Anaesth Intensive Care 2001;29:463–72.

[14] Landry DW, Levin HR, Gallant EM, et al. Vasopressin pressor hypersensitivity in vasodilatory septic shock. Crit Care Med 1997;25(8):1279–82.

[15] Holmes CL, Landry DW, Granton JT. Science review: vasopressin and the cardiovascular system: part 2—clinical physiology. Crit Care 2004;8(1):15–23.

[16] Argenziano M, Choudhri AF, Oz MC, et al. A prospective randomized trial of arginine vasopressin in the treatment of vasodilatory shock after left ventricular assist device placement. Circulation 1997;96(9 Suppl):II-286– 90.

[17] Argenziano M, Chen JM, Cullinane S, et al. Arginine vasopressin in the management of vasodilatory hypotension after cardiac transplantation. J Heart Lung Transplant 1999;18(8):814–7.

[18] Morales DL, Gregg D, Helman DN, et al. Arginine vasopressin in the treatment of 50 patients with postcardiotomy vasodilatory shock. Ann Thorac Surg 2000;69(1):102–6.

[19] Gold J, Cullinane S, Chen J, et al. Vasopressin in the treatment of milrinone-induced hypotension in severe heart failure [abstract A11]. Am J Cardiol 2000;85(4):506–8.

[20] Dunser MW, Mayr AJ, Ulmer H, et al. The effects of vasopressin on systemic hemodynamics in catecholamine-resistant septic and postcardiotomy shock: a retrospective analysis. Anesth Analg 2001;93(1):7–13.

[21] Masetti P, Murphy SF, Kouchoukos NT. Vasopressin therapy for vasoplegic syndrome following cardiopulmonary bypass. J Card Surg 2002;17(6):485–9.

[22] Dunser MW, Mayr AJ, Stallinger A, et al. Cardiac performance during vasopressin infusion in postcardiotomy shock. Intensive Care Med 2002;28(6):746–51.

[23] Jolly S, Newton G, Horlick E, et al. Effect of vasopressin on hemodynamics in patients with refractory cardiogenic shock complicating acute myocardial infarction. Am J Cardiol 2005; 96(12):1617–20.

[24] Morales DL, Garrido MJ, Madigan JD, et al. A double-blind randomized trial: prophylactic vasopressin reduces hypotension after cardiopulmonary bypass. Ann Thorac Surg 2003;75(3): 926–30.
[25] Sharshar T, Blanchard A, Paillard M, et al. Circulating vasopressin concentrations in septic shock. Crit Care Med 2003;31(6):1752–8.
[26] Landry DW, Levin HR, Gallant EM, et al. Vasopressin deficiency contributes to the vasodilation of septic shock. Circulation 1997;95(5):1122–5.
[27] Mohring J, Glanzer K, Maciel Jr JA, et al. Greatly enhanced pressor response to antidiuretic hormone in patients with impaired cardiovascular reflexes due to idiopathic orthostatic hypotension. J Cardiovasc Pharmacol 1980;2(4):367–76.
[28] Ebert TJ, Cowley Jr AW, Skelton M. Vasopressin reduces cardiac function and augments cardiopulmonary baroreflex resistance increases in man. J Clin Invest 1986;77(4):1136–42.
[29] Sharshar T, Carlier R, Blanchard A, et al. Depletion of neurohypophyseal content of vasopressin in septic shock. Crit Care Med 2002;30:497–500.
[30] Vincent JL. Endocrine support in the critically ill. Crit Care Med 2002;30:702–3.
[31] Malay MB, Ashton Jr RC, Landry DW, et al. Low-dose vasopressin in the treatment of vasodilatory septic shock. J Trauma 1999;47(4):699–703.
[32] Holmes CL, Walley KR, Chittock DR, et al. The effects of vasopressin on hemodynamics and renal function in severe septic shock: a case series. Intensive Care Med 2001;27(8):1416–21.
[33] Tsuneyoshi I, Yamada H, Kakihana Y, et al. Hemodynamic and metabolic effects of low-dose vasopressin infusions in vasodilatory septic shock. Crit Care Med 2001;29(3):487–93.
[34] Patel BM, Chittock DR, Russell JA, et al. Beneficial effects of short-term vasopressin infusion during severe septic shock. Anesthesiology 2002;96(3):576–82.
[35] Hall LG, Oyen LJ, Taner CB, et al. Fixed-dose vasopressin compared with titrated dopamine and norepinephrine as initial vasopressor therapy for septic shock. Pharmacotherapy 2004; 24(8):1002–12.
[36] Martikainen TJ, Tenhunen JJ, Uusaro A, et al. The effects of vasopressin on systemic and splanchnic hemodynamics and metabolism in endotoxin shock. Anesth Analg 2003;97(6): 1756–63.
[37] Asfar P, Hauser B, Ivanyi Z, et al. Low-dose terlipressin during long-term hyperdynamic porcine endotoxemia: effects on hepatosplanchnic perfusion, oxygen exchange, and metabolism. Crit Care Med 2005;33(2):373–80.
[38] Malay MB, Ashton JL, Dahl K, et al. Heterogeneity of the vasoconstrictor effect of vasopressin in septic shock. Crit Care Med 2004;32(6):1327–31.
[39] Knotzer H, Maier S, Dunser MW, et al. Arginine vasopressin does not alter mucosal tissue oxygen tension and oxygen supply in an acute endotoxemic pig model. Intensive Care Med 2006;32(1):170–4.
[40] Sun Q, Dimopoulos G, Nguyen DN, et al. Low-dose vasopressin in the treatment of septic shock in sheep. Am J Respir Crit Care Med 2003;168(4):481–6.
[41] van Haren FM, Rozendaal FW, van der Hoeven JG. The effect of vasopressin on gastric perfusion in catecholamine-dependent patients in septic shock. Chest 2003;124(6):2256–60.
[42] Klinzing S, Simon M, Reinhart K, et al. High-dose vasopressin is not superior to norepinephrine in septic shock. Crit Care Med 2003;31(11):2646–50.
[43] Morelli A, Rocco M, Conti G, et al. Effects of terlipressin on systemic and regional haemodynamics in catecholamine-treated hyperkinetic septic shock. Intensive Care Med 2004;30(4): 597–604.
[44] Dunser MW, Mayr AJ, Ulmer H, et al. Arginine vasopressin in advanced vasodilatory shock: a prospective, randomized, controlled study. Circulation 2003;107(18):2313–9.
[45] Edwards RM, Trizna W, Kinter LB. Renal microvascular effects of vasopressin and vasopressin antagonists. Am J Physiol 1989;256(2 Pt 2):F274–8.
[46] Obritsch MD, Jung R, Fish DN, et al. Effects of continuous vasopressin infusion in patients with septic shock. Ann Pharmacother 2004;38(7–8):1117–22.
[47] Kahn JM, Kress JP, Hall JB. Skin necrosis after extravasation of low-dose vasopressin administered for septic shock. Crit Care Med 2002;30(8):1899–901.

[48] Dunser MW, Mayr AJ, Tur A, et al. Ischemic skin lesions as a complication of continuous vasopressin infusion in catecholamine-resistant vasodilatory shock: incidence and risk factors. Crit Care Med 2003;31(5):1394–8.

[49] Luckner G, Dunser MW, Jochberger S, et al. Arginine vasopressin in 316 patients with advanced vasodilatory shock. Crit Care Med 2005;33(11):2659–66.

[50] Dunser MW, Fries DR, Schobersberger W, et al. Does arginine vasopressin influence the coagulation system in advanced vasodilatory shock with severe multiorgan dysfunction syndrome? Anesth Analg 2004;99(1):201–6.

[51] Bucher M, Kees F, Taeger K, et al. Cytokines down-regulate alpha1-adrenergic receptor expression during endotoxemia. Crit Care Med 2003;31(2):566–71.

[52] Dellinger RP, Carlet JM, Masur H, et al. Surviving Sepsis Campaign guidelines for management of severe sepsis and septic shock. Crit Care Med 2004;32(3):858–73.

[53] Jochberger S, Mayr VD, Luckner G, et al. Serum vasopressin concentrations in critically ill patients. Crit Care Med 2006;34(2):293–9.

[54] Dunser MW, Hasibeder WR, Wenzel V, et al. Endocrinologic response to vasopressin infusion in advanced vasodilatory shock. Crit Care Med 2004;32(6):1266–71.

[55] Duenser MW, Hasibeder WR. Dear vasopressin, where is your place in septic shock? Crit Care 2005;9(2):134–5.

[56] Lin IY, Ma HP, Lin AC, et al. Low plasma vasopressin/norepinephrine ratio predicts septic shock. Am J Emerg Med 2005;23(6):718–24.

ELSEVIER
SAUNDERS

Crit Care Clin 22 (2006) 199–219

CRITICAL
CARE
CLINICS

Contemporary Issues in the Pharmacologic Management of Acute Heart Failure

Tien M.H. Ng, PharmD[a,*], Amardeep K. Singh, MD[b], Joseph F. Dasta, MSc[c], David Feldman, MD, PhD[d], Alexandre Mebazaa, MD, PhD[e]

[a]*Department of Pharmacy, University of Southern California, 1985 Zonal Avenue, Los Angeles, CA 90033, USA*
[b]*Department of Internal Medicine, University of Southern California, 2020 Zonal Avenue, IRD 6th floor, Los Angeles, CA 90033, USA*
[c]*College of Pharmacy, The Ohio State University, 500 West 12th Avenue, Columbus, OH 43210-1291, USA*
[d]*Departments of Medicine/Cardiology & Physiology and Cell Biology, The Ohio State University, Suite 200, Davis Heart & Lung Institute, 473 West 12th Avenue Columbus, OH 43210-1252, USA*
[e]*Department of Anesthesiology and Critical Care Medicine, Hopitale Laribiosiere, Paris, France*

Heart failure has emerged as a disease with significant public health implications. There are about 5 million heart failure patients in the United States, and more than 400,000 new cases are diagnosed annually [1]. These patients generate 12 million to 15 million office visits each year for heart failure [2]. More than 266,000 patients die of heart failure each year [3]. The risk of death within 5 years of diagnosis is greater than 50%. Despite these data, funding for heart failure research has been limited. Although $28.7 million was spent on research for heart failure, $132 million was spent for lung cancer research, a disease with a population only 8% the size of patients with heart failure.

Epidemiology of acute heart failure

Acute heart failure (AHF) accounts for 5% to 10% of all hospital admissions and results in 6.5 million hospital days each year [2]. Seventy-six percent of

* Corresponding author.
E-mail address: tienng@usc.edu (T.M.H. Ng).

doi:10.1016/j.ccc.2006.02.008 ***criticalcare.theclinics.com***

patients are older than 65 years old, and Medicare is the payer in 70% of these admissions. Heart failure is the most common diagnosis for patients on Medicare. From 1993–2001, hospital discharges for heart failure as a primary diagnosis increased from 893,300 to 1,019,553 [4]. Another 2 million admissions are accounted for by patients with a secondary diagnosis of heart failure. Other studies have estimated 4 million hospitalizations in the United States with primary or secondary discharge diagnosis of heart failure [5]. A registry of nearly 500,000 hospitalized heart failure patients in 2003 revealed that secondary heart failure patients accounted for 75% of all cases [6]; this emphasizes the importance of patients developing heart failure after admission for another condition.

Despite improved availability of sophisticated diagnostic techniques and use of modern therapies, hospital length of stay for patients with AHF has remained fairly constant since 1996 at approximately 4 to 6 days [4,7]. Patients with a secondary diagnosis of heart failure have longer lengths of stay, averaging 9.5 days [6]. In contrast to the United States, the average length of stay in Europe is 11 days, with 6% requiring more than 1 week in the hospital [8].

The in-hospital mortality rate of patients admitted for AHF averages 4% (range 2.1–22%) [7,9]. Patients with AHF as a secondary diagnosis have double the mortality rate (average 8%) [6]. Patients requiring admission to an ICU have a mortality rate averaging 10.6% [7]. The ability to predict in-hospital mortality using clinical variables has been shown by analyzing data from a large retrospective database [10]. The three primary admission parameters associated with the highest mortality, in order of predictive value, were blood urea nitrogen greater than 43 mg/dL, systolic blood pressure less than 115 mm Hg, and serum creatinine greater than 2.76 mg/dL. It may be possible to use these readily available clinical parameters to classify patients into high, intermediate, and low risk of death and lead to more efficient and effective use of hospital resources.

Pathophysiologic considerations in acute heart failure

The pathophysiologic model for heart failure has evolved from hemodynamics to a more complex appreciation for the disease, which includes recognition of the roles of neurohormonal activation and renal disease [11]. The hemodynamic model of heart failure focuses on the physiologic responses to and consequences of diminished cardiac output and elevated filling pressures. Despite its limitations, the hemodynamic model of heart failure continues to guide AHF therapy [12].

The neurohormonal model of heart failure takes the hemodynamic model further by linking the progressive decline in ventricular function to the compensatory response to the decrease in cardiac output. The original neurohormonal model implicated four systems: sympathetic nervous system, renin-angiotensin-aldosterone, endothelin, and vasopressin [13,14]. Activation of these systems leads to vasoconstriction, increased intravascular volume, and increased inotropy to increase cardiac output and maintain perfusion to vital organs. Although acute hemodynamic improvement is achieved, activation of these systems contributes to an increased preload, increased afterload, increased myocardial workload, proarrhythmia (secondary to increase in intracellular calcium), decreased lusitropy, and trophic effects. All these effects lead to a vicious cycle of accelerated myocyte death and pathologic remodeling, further decline in cardiac function, and greater activation of the neurohormonal systems.

The cardiorenal model is based on the mounting evidence for a relationship between renal disease and heart failure. In AHF, renal disease is a comorbid illness in approximately one third of patients [7]. Elevated admission serum creatinine and blood urea nitrogen and diminished estimated creatinine clearance have been shown to be poor prognostic markers [10]. In addition, treatment of AHF commonly is complicated by acute renal insufficiency. Drugs such as diuretics and vasodilators can impair renal filtration through hypotension, hypoperfusion, and potentially neurohormonal activation [15,16]. This complication of drug therapy is clinically important because hospitalized patients experiencing acute renal insufficiency are more likely to experience longer lengths of stay and increased morbidity and mortality [17]. Renal failure also is a common cause of acute decompensation. The neurohormonal and cardiorenal models are now important considerations in the pharmacotherapeutic management of AHF. As understanding of the pathophysiologic processes in AHF continues to grow, the role of other systems and components of cardiac function, such as inflammation, cellular and molecular alterations, and gene expression, will become more defined.

Demographics, clinical presentation, and diagnostics

Insight into the demographics of heart failure patients presenting in acute decompensation has largely been derived from registries. Based on the Acute Decompensated Heart Failure National Registry (ADHERE) registry, patients are older (mean age 75 years), are more often female (52%), and present with significant comorbidities (coronary artery disease in 58%, hypertension in 74%, diabetes mellitus in 44%, and renal insufficiency in 31%) [7]. Most patients have systolic dysfunction (57%), but there are a significant number with preserved left ventricular function (43%). The initial workup of these patients requires clinical evaluation and appropriate laboratory and diagnostic assessments.

Signs and symptoms of AHF are in part the result of either congestive symptoms or a low perfusion state. Right-sided failure results in systemic findings, such as diuretic-resistant shortness of breath secondary to elevated pulmonary pressures, jugular venous distention, hepatojugular reflux, peripheral or intestinal edema, and hepatic congestion (hepatomegaly or hepatic insufficiency). Left-sided failure manifests as pulmonary congestion, rales, positive S_3 heart sound, worsening orthopnea, and paroxysmal nocturnal dyspnea. Hypoperfusion contributes to altered end-organ function, including brain, liver, and kidneys. General symptoms include dyspnea, fatigue, difficulty concentrating, and decreased exercise tolerance. It has been reported that greater than 90% of patients present with some degree of congestion [7]. Resolution of these signs and symptoms remains an integral part of managing and monitoring these patients.

Diagnostics

B-type natriuretic peptide (BNP) is synthesized primarily by ventricular myocytes in response to wall stretch. Assays have been developed for determination of plasma levels of the active compound and the degradation product N-terminal proBNP (NT-proBNP). NT-proBNP has the potential diagnostic advantage of greater plasma level stability secondary to a longer half-life of 118 minutes compared with 18 minutes for BNP (in normal renal function). More recently, BNP and NT-proBNP are being used for diagnosis of heart failure. Studies have shown that plasma BNP or NT-proBNP concentrations correlate positively with worsening New York Heart Association functional class in an ambulatory setting [18,19]. Other studies show a role for obtaining an admission BNP or NT-proBNP concentration in the rapid diagnosis of heart failure in an emergency department and for aiding in diagnosing and ruling out a cardiac etiology for dyspnea [18,20–25].

BNP concentrations are generally higher in ventricular systolic dysfunction compared with diastolic dysfunction [26]. The role of BNP in diagnosing diastolic dysfunction remains to be determined. There also is evidence to support a role for BNP assessment in prognostication and risk stratification. Higher concentrations are associated with worse clinical outcomes after adjustment for other markers of disease severity, such as functional class and ejection fraction [27]. The role of serial BNP and NT-proBNP monitoring for guiding therapy remains controversial, however, because supporting data from large prospective trials are lacking [28–33].

The current cut-points for ruling out a cardiac etiology for dyspnea are less than 100 pg/mL or less than 300 pg/mL for NT-proBNP [34]. One must remain cognizant, however, that interpretation of BNP concentrations may be confounded by comorbid illnesses (Table 1). Because recombinant BNP (nesiritide) is identical in structure to endogenous BNP, caution must be taken when interpreting levels during the use of nesiritide. Blood for BNP concentration should be taken after nesiritide has been discontinued for 2 hours (elimination half-life approximately 18 minutes in normal renal function). In contrast, the NT-proBNP assay is unaffected by concomitant nesiritide therapy.

Currently, BNP or NT-proBNP assays are useful as an adjunctive tool to aid in the rapid diagnosis of heart failure in patients presenting with dyspnea, especially when a patient does not have a previous history of cardiac disease. It should not be used in place of a thorough clinical assessment. Further investigation is needed

Table 1
Factors affecting interpretation of plasma B-type natriuretic peptide level

Influencing factor	Effect on B-type natriuretic peptide level
Increasing age	↑
Female gender	↑
Renal insufficiency	↑
Pulmonary disease	↑
Hyperthyroidism	↑
Glucocorticoid use	↑
Hepatic cirrhosis	↑
Subarachnoid hemorrhage	↑
Obesity	↓

before routine serial monitoring can be advocated confidently. The evidence for a role of BNP assays has been reviewed more extensively elsewhere [35,36].

An electrocardiogram should be obtained in all patients. The electrocardiogram is useful for identifying or ruling out potential etiologic factors, such as arrhythmias and ischemia. It also is helpful in identifying the presence of underlying cardiac conditions that may contribute or reflect the heart failure syndrome, such as myocarditis, hypertrophy, or myocardial strain.

A chest radiograph is obtained to provide information regarding pulmonary congestion and cardiac structure (cardiomegaly or dilation). Chest radiography in heart failure often reveals cardiac enlargement with an increase in the cardiothoracic ratio. As left atrial pressure increases, cephalization, or vascular redistribution to the upper lung lobes, occurs. Worsening congestion manifests with Kerly B lines, lines perpendicular the pleura that are caused by fluid along interlobuolar septa. In severe congestion, alveolar edema obscures vessel margins, and pleural effusions may cause obscuring of the costophrenic and cardiophrenic angles.

Echocardiography is helpful in the diagnosis and etiologic assessment of cardiac dysfunction in heart failure. Segmental or global ventricular function, chamber size, pulmonary artery pressure, valvular function, and hemodynamics all may aid in the diagnosis and etiology of heart failure.

In complex or refractory patients, pulmonary artery catheters may be employed to clarify cardiac hemodynamics. In most AHF patients, an elevated pulmonary capillary wedge pressure (PCWP) and reduced cardiac output are seen. Pulmonary artery catheters also can aid in diagnosis and treatment monitoring in AHF, although their routine use has not been shown to improve outcomes [37].

Hemodynamic subsets

Based on the clinical assessment and diagnostic evaluations, AHF patients can be classified into hemodynamic subsets (Fig. 1) [12]. These subsets often are used as a guide to determine the therapeutic approach based on hemodynamic goals. Although choosing pharmacologic therapy based solely on the subset a

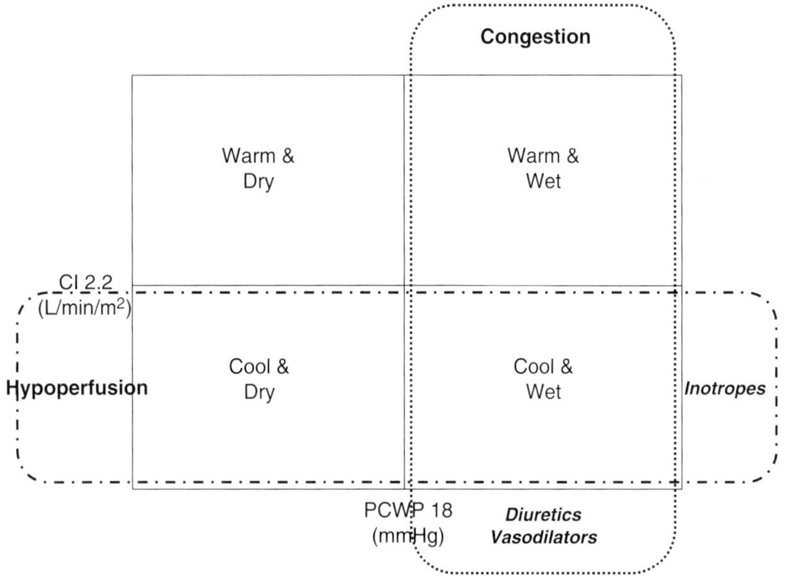

Fig. 1. Hemodynamic subsets in acute heart failure. CI, cardiac index.

patient falls into is too simplistic, the principles of targeting congestion and hypoperfusion continue to apply to the current paradigm of AHF management.

Current pharmacologic strategies

The paradigm for managing acute decompensation has remained relatively constant since the 1990s. Limited understanding of acute pathophysiologic processes, coupled with a lack of new therapeutic agents, forced the focus of therapy to remain solely on improvement in hemodynamics with little regard for how it was achieved. This situation may explain why length of stay has remained stationary. More recently, recognition of in-hospital prognostic indicators, such as hyponatremia, renal insufficiency, and hypotension, has led to a re-evaluation of the hemodynamic paradigm. In addition, emerging data show that depending on which hemodynamic parameter is targeted and how it is treated, prognostic implications can vary. Post hoc analysis suggests that targeting cardiac output in hospitalized heart failure patients does not modify outcomes, whereas reducing ventricular filling pressures is associated with a survival benefit [38]. Similarly, it is known that routine use of conventional positive inotropes to augment cardiac output is associated with detrimental outcomes despite hemodynamic improvement [39–42]. Future paradigms for AHF must take into account modification of the disease pathophysiology and hemodynamics.

The current goals of therapy should be to (1) identify and treat the underlying etiology or precipitating factors of acute decompensation, (2) relieve symptoms

Table 2
Common precipitating causes of acute heart failure

Cardiac	Metabolic	Patient
Acute ischemia	Anemia	Dietary/fluid noncompliance
Uncontrolled hypertension	Hyperthyroidism/thyrotoxicosis	Medication noncompliance
Pulmonary embolus	Pregnancy	Offending medications
Arrhythmia	Infection	(NSAIDs, COX-2 inhibitors,
Myocarditis		steroids, lithium, β-blockers,
Valvular dysfunction		calcium channel blockers,
Endocarditis		antiarrhythmics, alcohol,
		thiazolidinediones)

Abbreviations: COX-2, cyclooxygenase-2; NSAIDs, nonsteroidal anti-inflammatory drugs.

rapidly, (3) normalize or improve hemodynamics, (4) initiate or optimize long-term oral medications known to improve prognosis and functionality, and (5) initiate patient education to reinforce the importance of adherence to lifestyle modifications and compliance with disease-modifying medications. With the advent of new pharmacologic therapies, it may be possible to include an additional goal of using pharmacologic agents in the acute setting that potentially modify the disease process in a beneficial manner acutely and long-term.

Some important concepts should be considered when addressing these goals. Common precipitating factors of acute decompensation are listed in Table 2. These must be managed to ensure optimal response to drugs. Rapid relief of symptoms and hemodynamic improvement are achieved by aggressive titration of medications to desired therapeutic responses and using rational drug combinations, such as diuretics and vasodilators for acute congestion. Disease-modifying long-term oral medications include angiotensin antagonists (angiotensin-converting enzyme inhibitors or angiotensin receptor blockers), β-blockers (metoprolol succinate, bisoprolol, or carvedilol), aldosterone antagonists (spironolactone or eplerenone), and possibly hydroxymethylglutaryl-coenzyme A reductase inhibitors (statins). Antiplatelets or anticoagulation therapy when clinically indicated also may modify outcomes. The common practice of routinely discontinuing β-blockers in all patients in acute decompensation should be discouraged. From a pathophysiologic standpoint, neurohormonal activation is most evident during acute decompensations, and it would be reasonable to anticipate that the need for cardioprotection would be greatest in these instances. In addition, the Carvedilol Prospective Randomized Cumulative Survival (COPERNICUS) study found the greatest benefit from carvedilol in New York Heart Association functional class IV patients was in the sickest subset presenting with low systolic blood pressures [43,44]. The comparative hemodynamic effects of intravenous agents used in AHF are outlined in Table 3.

Diuretics

Diuretics are the most commonly used drugs for providing symptomatic relief from pulmonary and peripheral congestion in mild to severe acute decompensated

Table 3
Comparative effects of common intravenous agents used in acute heart failure

	CO	PCWP	SVR	BP	HR	MVO_2	Arrhythmias	Neurohormonal activation	Mortality
Diuretics	↑/↓/0	↓	?	↓	0	?	↑	↑	?
Nitroglycerin	↑	↓↓	↓	↓↓	↑/0	↓	0	↑?	?
Nitroprusside	↑	↓↓↓	↓↓↓	↓↓↓	↑	?	0	↑?	?
Nesiritide	↑	↓↓	↓↓	↓↓	0	?	0	↓	?
Dobutamine	↑↑	↓/0	↓/0	↓/0	↑↑	↑	↑	↑	↑
Milrinone	↑↑	↓↓	↓	↓	↑	↑	↑	↑	↑

Abbreviations: BP, blood pressure; CO, cardiac output; HR, heart rate; MVO_2, myocardial oxygen consumption; 0, no or little change; ?, unknown.

heart failure. Loop diuretics (furosemide, bumetanide, or torsemide) block the sodium-potassium-chloride transporter in the ascending loop of Henle [45,46]. Because of their potent natriuretic effects, rapid onset, and short duration of action, loop diuretics are a mainstay of therapy in moderate to severe heart failure. Thiazide diuretics (hydrochlorothiazide, metolazone, or chlorthalidone) act at the distal tubule of the nephron to block the sodium-chloride transporter and often are used in the treatment of mild congestive heart failure. Thiazides are not as effective at achieving diuresis compared with loop diuretics, however. Thiazides usually are reserved for combination therapy with loop diuretics to provide a synergistic response in patients refractory to loop diuretics alone [45,46]. Potassium-sparing diuretics, such as amiloride and triamterene, act at the distal tubule sodium channels of the nephron. Spironolactone (and eplerenone), another potassium diuretic, is a specific inhibitor of aldosterone and acts to promote natriuresis. Potassium-sparing agents are weak diuretics and have a limited role in AHF.

Loop diuretics can be administered as intermittent boluses or by a continuous infusion (Table 4). Continuous infusions use the concept that diuresis is achieved only after a certain threshold of drug is active at the nephron, but further increases in dose have little additional effect. Limited data suggest that continuous infusions are more effective at increasing urine output [47–50]. In addition, continuous infusions may reduce the risk of adverse effects with high-dose diuretics. Before the use of any diuretic, a diet low in sodium content or sodium restriction must be implemented for effective diuresis. Patients receiving diuretics must be monitored

Table 4
Comparison of intravenous loop diuretics

	Onset of action (min)	Peak (min)	Duration of action (h)	Relative potency	Intermittent bolus dosing (mg)	Continuous infusion dosing (bolus/infusion)
Furosemide	2–5	30	6	40	20–200+	20–40/2.5–10
Torsemide	<10	60	6–12	20	10–100	20/2–5
Bumetanide	2–3	15–30	4–6	0.5	1–10	1–4/0.5–1
Ethacrynic acid	5–15	15–180	2–7		0.5–1 mg/kg/dose up to 100 mg/dose	

frequently for achievement of adequate urine output and indicators of volume depletion. Because of the potential implications of inducing acute renal insufficiency, monitoring for and holding diuretics at the first indication of prerenal azotemia is important. Patients also should be monitored for metabolic alkalosis, hyponatremia, hypokalemia, hypomagnesemia, and hyperuricemia [51].

Although diuretics are currently the most effective means for removing excess intravascular fluid volume, adverse reactions should be considered. Diuretic administration results in an acute reduction in glomerular filtration; this may reflect a decrease in intravascular volume and indicate reduced renal perfusion, but is likely also a complication of increased neurohormonal activation. The renin-angiotensin-aldosterone system is activated by diuretics [15]. This fact may have implications on long-term disease progression. In addition, diuretics exacerbate hyponatremia and other electrolyte abnormalities that influence heart failure prognosis and proarrhythmic risk. These considerations are providing the impetus for development of new diuretic, natriuretic, and aquaretic agents.

Vasodilators (nitroglycerin, nitroprusside)

Vasodilators have become the therapeutic class of choice for most AHF patients presenting with moderate to severe congestion. The intravenous agents included in this class are nitroglycerin, nitroprusside, and nesiritide (discussed separately). Vasodilators are contraindicated in patients with significant outflow obstruction, volume-dependent cardiac filling, or shock. A more recent study suggests, however, that nitroprusside may be beneficial if used carefully in patients with AHF secondary to severe aortic stenosis [52]. Nitroprusside also is indicated for acute mitral regurgitation secondary to papillary rupture—post myocardial infarction or acute aortic insufficiency. In all cases of aortic stenosis and aortic or mitral insufficiency, vasodilators must be used with great caution.

Nitroglycerin is metabolized, in part, to nitric oxide, which induces vasorelaxation through the generation of cyclic guanosine monophosphate. Nitroglycerin is a potent venodilator, with increasing arterial vasodilatory effects as dosage is increased. The dose-dependent pharmacology of nitroglycerin has important clinical implications because venous and arterial vasodilation is desirable for relieving elevated filling pressures of congested patients. One study suggests that, on average, doses greater than 120 μg/min are required to confer significant reductions in PCWP [53]. Frequent assessments for the need to adjust doses also are required because tolerance to the effects of nitroglycerin may be evident within 12 hours of initiating a continuous infusion [53]. The clinical implications of using inadequate doses of intravenous nitroglycerin were shown in the Vasodilation in the Management of Acute Congestive Heart failure trial, in which a mean nitroglycerin dose of only 42 μg/min in patients with a pulmonary artery catheter was inferior to nesiritide in reducing PCWP at 1 and 3 hours [18,54]. No prospective mortality studies have been conducted with nitroglycerin in AHF. The most common adverse event reported with nitroglycerin is headache. In addition to monitoring for PCWP response, patients receiving nitroglycerin require monitoring for hypotension, reflex tachycardia, and headache.

Nitroprusside is a complex of iron, five cyanide moieties, and a nitroso group. It is metabolized rapidly in red blood cells to release its components. Similar to nitroglycerin, nitroprusside acts as a nitroso donor, which leads to the formation of nitric oxide and vascular smooth muscle relaxation. In contrast to nitroglycerin, nitroprusside is a balanced venous and arterial vasodilator at all dosages. Titratability of nitroprusside is the major advantage of this agent. Its effects are evident within 30 seconds of initiation and persist for only 3 minutes after discontinuation. There are limited controlled clinical data for nitroprusside in AHF, and no studies have evaluated its effects on mortality. As with nitroglycerin, nitroprusside requires strict monitoring of blood pressure and heart rate. An arterial catheter generally is used with nitroprusside. Its use must be limited in patients with renal insufficiency, secondary to accumulation of thiocyanate or cyanide, and in heart failure with concordant hypotension. Nitroprusside also has been implicated in coronary steal, the phenomenon of preferential dilation of patent nondiseased coronary arteries, which could exacerbate underlying ischemic heart disease.

Nesiritide

Recombinant BNP or nesiritide was the first compound developed for AHF based on a greater understanding of the pathophysiologic processes that contribute to the development, sustenance, and progression of the disease. BNP is a naturally occurring neurohormone that is synthesized and released from the ventricles in response to stretch or increased filling pressures. Physiologically, release of BNP results in vasodilation, natriuresis, and antagonism of the effects of angiotensin II.

Nesiritide's beneficial effects on hemodynamics, neurohormonal activation, and symptoms have been shown in several randomized clinical trials, which included more than 1000 patients randomized to the drug [54–58]. Compared with placebo, nesiritide reduces PCWP, right atrial pressure, and systemic vascular resistance within 1 hour of administration of a bolus dose followed by a fixed-dose continuous infusion [55,56]; this is accompanied by an increase in cardiac output and stroke volume index. Usually no significant change in heart rate is experienced. The beneficial hemodynamic effects are sustained for 24 hours without evidence for tachyphylaxis [54–56]. These hemodynamic benefits are associated with improvement in symptoms of dyspnea and fatigue [54,56]. Compared with intravenous nitroglycerin, nesiritide was shown to be more effective at reducing PCWP early (15 minutes to 3 hours); however, the difference was not significant at 24 hours [54]. No difference in improvement in dyspnea scores has been shown between nesiritide and intravenous nitroglycerin. One criticism of the pivotal trial comparing nesiritide with nitroglycerin was the relatively low median dose of nitroglycerin used. Higher dose nitroglycerin (>100 μg/min) in terms of efficacy and safety remains equivocal. Nesiritide also is not associated with any increased risk of ventricular ectopy and compares favorably with dobutamine in this regard [57].

Nesiritide is indicated for patients in acutely decompensated heart failure with dyspnea at rest or with minimal exertion. Nesiritide is primarily a vasodilator and should not be used as monotherapy to achieve diuresis. Nesiritide should be avoided in patients with evidence of shock (systolic blood pressure < 90 mm Hg) or in patients in whom vasodilators are contraindicated (eg, low cardiac filling pressures or significant left ventricular outflow obstruction). The recommended dose regimen is a 2 μg/kg bolus, followed by a continuous infusion of 0.01 μg/kg/min, although reducing the bolus dose to 1 μg/kg and initiating the infusion at 0.005 μg/kg/min have been used clinically. The dose may be titrated up by 0.005 μg/kg/min no more frequently than every 3 hours, to a maximum approved dose of 0.03 μg/kg/min. Most patients do not require a dose greater than 0.01 μg/kg/min to achieve hemodynamic improvement. In patients with borderline low systolic blood pressures, the bolus dose may be withheld, although this is an empiric practice. The infusion usually is maintained for 24 hours, but may be continued if necessary, although infusions greater than 48 hours are rarely indicated.

Nesiritide's place in AHF therapy remains to be firmly defined. Based on its unique pharmacology and demonstrated benefits, nesiritide could be regarded as a first-line agent (in combination with diuretics) for most patients presenting in moderate to severe decompensation. Two publications have questioned the safety of the drug, however [59,60]. In both instances, meta-analyses were conducted using data from previously conducted clinical trials. The first meta-analysis showed an association between randomization to nesiritide and an increased risk of experiencing an increase in serum creatinine at any time 30 days after exposure. The second analysis suggested nesiritide was associated with an increased risk of 30-day mortality. Both analyses contained severe limitations, including lack of adjustment for numerous confounding variables and use of nonadjudicated raw data. Subsequent analyses of pooled data from all clinical trials have shown no clear signal that nesiritide is associated with an increased risk of death [58,61]. Post-hoc analyses show no indication that patients who experienced an increase in serum creatinine had a worse outcome [62]. Despite the provocative meta-analyses, there are currently no prospective outcome data with nesiritide (or any other vasodilator) in AHF. Ongoing prospective clinical trials are needed to clarify nesiritide's safety and place in therapy.

Inotropes

Based on the hemodynamic model, a decrease in cardiac contractility contributes to hypoperfusion of vital organs. Consequently, positive inotropes were used to increase cardiac output in an effort to resolve symptoms. Although short-term improvement in hemodynamics and symptoms may be seen, these effects are achieved at the expense of an increased risk of worsening heart failure and mortality [39,41,63]. The exception is digoxin, which exhibits weak inotropic and neurohormonal properties [64]. Digoxin has no defined role in AHF, however, and although it has been shown to decrease hospitalizations when used at low doses on a long-term basis, there are no data to support a beneficial effect when used emergently.

Inotropic agents act via stimulation of β-adrenergic-induced cyclic adenosine monophosphate (cAMP) production (dobutamine, dopamine) or inhibition of phosphodiesterase III leading to a decrease in cAMP breakdown (milrinone). An increase in cAMP leads to an increase in available intracellular calcium and greater contractile force generation by myocytes. The increase in intracellular calcium is associated with increased proarrhythmic risk and myocardial oxygen demand. Catecholamine inotropes may have a direct toxic effect on myocytes, and stimulation of hibernating myocardium may accelerate myocyte apoptosis [65,66].

As a consequence, inotropes should not be used routinely in AHF. Current recommended indications have been limited to the following: (1) cardiogenic shock; (2) patients refractory to optimal doses of diuretics and angiotensin-converting enzyme inhibitors, especially when associated with hypotension and renal failure; (3) bridging to a definitive treatment, such as cardiac transplant or revascularization; and (4) palliative treatment for patients with severe heart failure who are not candidates for definitive treatment and in which case quality of life is the focus, rather than prolongation of life [63]. For palliative patients, the decision to use inotropes should be made by the physician and the informed patient. The choice of inotrope depends on clinician preference, but should incorporate an understanding of the pharmacologic differences (see Table 3). Phosphodiesterase inhibitors also are potent vasodilators and must be used judiciously in patients with borderline low systolic blood pressures and renal insufficiency. These agents also have a relatively long elimination half-life, reducing their acute titratability. In addition, β-blockers may accentuate the hemodynamic response to milrinone, whereas they antagonize the therapeutic effects of inotropes using β-adrenergic signaling, such as dobutamine [66].

Pharmacologic agents on the horizon

The myriad of limitations that exist with the current pharmacotherapeutic options for the management of AHF have been outlined previously. Newer compounds and treatment modalities have been developed or are in development. These therapies hold the promise of achieving positive hemodynamic outcomes without adversely affecting the underlying pathophysiology, and some have the potential for improvement in morbidity and mortality.

Vasopressin receptor antagonists

Vasopressin was implicated in the original neurohormonal model of heart failure. Vasopressin exerts its detrimental effects in heart failure through activation of V1a receptors in the vasculature and heart and V2 receptors in the kidneys [67]. V1a stimulation results in vasoconstriction, exacerbation of myocardial ischemia, and modulation of cardiac remodeling. V2 stimulation results in expression of aquaporin channels on the apical surface of the renal collecting ducts and subsequent retention of free water. The clinical utility of dual blockade of V1a and V2 receptors has been evaluated in AHF patients presenting with volume overload [68–70]. In a double-blind, placebo-controlled trial, 142 patients with symptomatic moderate to severe heart failure (cardiac index $\leq$2.8 L/min/m^2 and PCWP $\geq$16 mm Hg) were randomized to a single dose of intravenous conivaptan or placebo [71]. Conivaptan was associated with dose-dependent reductions in PCWP and increases in urine output over 12 hours, with peak effects at 3 to 6 hours. Serum sodium increased, showing an aquaretic effect of these agents as opposed to the natriuretic effect of conventional diuretics. The role of dual (conivaptan) and selective (tolvaptan) vasopressin receptor antagonists for heart failure is expected to be defined by ongoing clinical trials such as Efficacy Vasopressin Antagonism in Heart Failure (EVEREST) and A Dose Evaluation of a Vasopressin Antagonist in CHF Patients Undergoing Exercise (ADVANCE). They are potentially useful in patients with hyponatremia and volume overload [70]. Conivaptan was approved more recently in the United States for euvolemic hyponatremia.

Calcium sensitizers

Inotropic agents still are required by patients with evidence of hypoperfusion refractory to other vasoactive therapies despite their detrimental effects on myocardial oxygen consumption, proarrhythmia, diastolic function, and outcomes. The paradigm of positive inotropism may change with the advent of drugs such as levosimendan, a novel dual mechanism compound for AHF. Currently approved for use in parts of Europe and Sweden, levosimendan is a potent positive inotrope and vasodilator. Its unique pharmacologic profile has been reviewed in detail elsewhere [72,73]. Briefly, levosimendan achieves an increase in myocyte contractile force generation through sensitization of troponin C to calcium, facilitating recruitment of more myofilaments during systole without increasing intracellular calcium concentrations or myocardial oxygen demand. Levosimendan exhibits calcium-dependent calcium sensitization, and it does not interfere with diastole. Levosimendan also is a significant vasodilator of pulmonary, cardiac, and peripheral vasculature through activation of adenosine triphosphate potassium channels. Activation of these channels, an effect analogous to ischemic preconditioning, also has been implicated in the safety of this agent in patients with ischemic heart disease. Levosimendan inhibits phosphodiesterase III at higher in vitro concentrations, which may or may not be relevant clinically.

There is now extensive clinical trial experience with levosimendan. Infusions of levosimendan for 24 hours have been associated with dose-dependent increases in cardiac output and reductions in PCWP. Small increases in heart rate have been observed. Earlier trials (Levosimendan Infusion versus Dobutamine

[LIDO]; Randomized Study on Safety and Effectiveness of Levosimendan in Patients with Left Ventriclar Failure Due to an Acute Myocadial Infarct [RUSSLAN]; and Calcium Sensitizer or Inotrope or None in Low Output Heart Failure [CASINO]) showed no significant risk of myocardial ischemia or proarrhythmia; however, the two most recent trials (Randomized Multicenter Evaluation of Intravenous Levosimendan Efficacy versus Placebo in the Short term Treatment of Decompensated Heart Failure study [REVIVE]-2 and Survival of Patients with Acute Heart Failure in Need of Intravenous Insotropic Support [SURVIVE]) indicate an increased risk of ventricular tachycardia and atrial fibrillation over placebo and a similar risk compared with dobutamine [74–77]. The utility of levosimendan as an inotrope or vasodilator for AHF remains to be clarified. Preliminary studies suggest it may be potentially useful in cardiac surgery, shock, and diastolic dysfunction.

Arial natriuretic peptides and adenosine-1 receptor antagonists

Two other novel drug classes being actively investigated for AHF are atrial natriuretic peptides (carperitide or ularitide) and adenosine-1 receptor antagonists. Atrial natriuretic peptides, similar to BNPs, offer the advantages of cardioprotection through antagonism of the renin-angiotensin-aldosterone system and sympathetic activation [78–82]. Hemodynamically, carperitide exerts effects similar to nesiritide [83,84]. Adenosine-1 receptors are located in the kidneys, predominantly on the afferent arteriole and proximal tubule. Activation of adenosine-1 receptors mediates renal function through vasoconstriction and sodium retention. Adenosine-1 receptor antagonists currently are being investigated for effectiveness as diuretics and renoprotection in AHF [16,85,86].

Ultrafiltration

Ultrafiltration or hemofiltration represents a nonpharmacologic modality for achieving effective intravascular volume removal in AHF [87,88]. It warrants mention because this modality can be considered an adjunct and potential replacement for high-dose diuretics. Advantages of a continuous, slow ultrafiltration strategy over conventional diuretics include the ability to correct electrolyte imbalances, improvement in diuretic responsiveness, and a reduction in neurohormonal activation. Ultrafiltration also exhibits a low propensity for intravascular volume depletion secondary to allowance of fluid mobilization from the interstitium. This modality currently is approved in the United States for short-term treatment of volume overload.

Pharmacoeconomic implications of acute heart failure

In 2005, the estimated direct and indirect cost of heart failure in the United States was $29.6 billion. This represents 7.1% of all cardiovascular diseases [3].

Fifty-two percent of these costs, or $15.4 billion, are for the hospitalized patient. Drug-related costs accounted for less than 10% of costs related to hospitalization. Because managing the hospitalized patient is a major determinant of total costs, ways to prevent admissions, reduce readmissions, and shorten the length of hospital stay are needed.

There are other issues regarding heart failure admissions that shed further insight into the financial implications of AHF. The Center for Medicare and Medicaid Services assigns a fixed reimbursement to a given diagnosis-related group (DRG). The break-even point for heart failure (DRG 127) occurs at 5 days [89]. In addition, the same amount of reimbursement is provided for heart failure patients regardless of the number of hospital readmissions within a 30-day period. The potential for significant financial loss to the institution exists for a patient readmitted within 30 days of an admission for heart failure. In one health care system of 1830 cases from eight hospitals in 2002, the average financial gain/loss per heart failure patient (DRG 127) varied according to disease severity. The least sick patient (n = 124) experienced a gain of $930, whereby the sickest patient (n = 108) resulted in an average loss to the hospital of $4291. Heart failure patients with renal failure generated a loss averaging $2503 (Vicas Gupta, personal communication). From another database of more than 16,000 admissions from 176 hospitals, the cost versus reimbursement revealed a mean loss of $2580 per case for patients with uncomplicated heart failure [90].

The average total hospital costs for patients with heart failure as a primary discharge diagnosis is $14,350 [6]. Patients with heart failure as a secondary discharge diagnosis had a 40% higher total hospital cost of $20,084. In another large database of patients with severe AHF from 1999–2003, defined as more than 3 days of inotropes and vasodilators, the total cost of hospitalization was $42,000 [5]. Despite the high costs associated with AHF, only a few studies evaluating the cost-effectiveness of therapies have been published. One study was a retrospective review of outcomes in 269 patients admitted to a heart failure unit from 1996–1999 receiving dobutamine compared with 60 patients receiving milrinone [91]. The mortality rate and other clinical outcomes were similar between the two groups; however, patients receiving milrinone had significantly higher direct drug costs compared with the dobutamine patients ($1855 versus $45). A cost-effectiveness analysis of a randomized trial that evaluated the clinical effects of levosimendan versus dobutamine administered for 24 hours in patients with AHF was performed [92]. There was an 11% absolute reduction in mortality at 6 months in patients receiving levosimendan; however, there were no differences in hospital stay or number of hospital readmissions. The incremental cost per life-year saved for levosimendan over a 3-year survival was 3205 Euros.

Four studies evaluated nesiritide because this agent has a high acquisition price compared with current therapies. One study developed an economic model from the hospital perspective using a Monte Carlo simulation of a clinical trial of patients with AHF randomized to dobutamine versus nesiritide [93]. In this study, nesiritide was more costly than dobutamine, but the increase in cost was fully offset by lower total hospital costs of an initial admission and significantly lower costs of readmissions for heart failure in the nesiritide group. The authors concluded that the cost-neutrality of nesiritide coupled with an increased survival of 0.53 years made nesiritide cost-effective compared with dobutamine. Conversely, an analysis using similar randomized clinical trial data in a decision tree model questioned the cost-effectiveness of nesiritide compared with dobutamine [94]. The authors concluded that when uncertainty over effectiveness is incorporated into the cost-effectiveness analyses, superiority of either nesiritide or dobutamine is possible. In a retrospective analysis, 108 patients receiving nesiritide for at least 12 hours during the first 48 hours of admission for AHF were matched to 108 patients not receiving nesiritide [95]. Patients receiving nesiritide had a significantly shorter length of stay in the critical care unit, required less use of inotropes and nitroglycerin, and experienced fewer episodes of atrial fibrillation and renal dysfunction. No resource use or costs were provided in this study. A follow-up study used a Markov model to estimate these costs [96]. They found the nesiritide cohort to be cost-effective primarily because of fewer readmissions. Most recently, a resource use analysis of a prospective, randomized study of nesiritide in the emergency department or observational unit was performed [97]. Using the hospital prospective, the acquisition cost for nesiritide was offset by a reduction in admissions and 30-day readmissions.

Institutional guidelines and protocols are being developed to standardize care and minimize excessive hospital costs. A guideline for the management of AHF has been published for use in hospitals that are part of a group purchasing organization [98]. An analysis of implementing this guideline compared with preguideline data revealed that although 5% more patients received nesiritide, there was a 44% decreased duration of intravenous vasoactive therapies, a 3-day shorter stay in the ICU, and nearly a 2-day decrease in hospital length of stay [99]. These findings suggest that guidelines and protocols may lead to optimal and less expensive care.

To understand better the costs and associated outcomes of current and future drug therapies for heart failure, it is suggested that a full economic evaluation be performed on future randomized clinical trials. This evaluation includes determining all relevant costs of drugs, such as acquisition cost; cost of preparation, distribution, and administration of the drug; costs associated with monitoring for safety and efficacy; cost of adverse drug events; and costs from various hospital departments, and relevant outcomes, such as short-term and long-term symptom resolution, length of stay in the ICU or critical care unit and hospital, incidence of renal dysfunction during therapy, use of other hospital resources, 30-day readmission rate, and in-hospital and long-term mortality rate.

Summary

AHF is an evolving syndrome that continues to be defined by ongoing studies and registries. It is associated with significant morbidity and mortality and places a huge economic burden on health care systems. Improved understanding of the underlying pathophysiologic processes has prompted interest into understanding the implications of current and future pharmacologic management strategies beyond hemodynamics. Diuretics, vasodilators, and inotropes remain the mainstays of therapy with several new classes of agents on the horizon. Clinicians should understand the rationale for use and limitations of each therapy to maximize benefit and cost-effectiveness, while minimizing the potential for adverse outcomes.

References

[1] Centers for Disease Control and Prevention. Heart failure fact sheet. Available at: www.cdc.gov/cvh/library/fs_heart_failure.htm.

[2] Bonow RO, Bennett S, Casey Jr DE, et al. ACC/AHA clinical performance measures for adults with chronic heart failure: a report of the American College of Cardiology/American Heart Association Task Force on Performance Measures (Writing Committee to Develop Heart Failure Clinical Performance Measures) endorsed by the Heart Failure Society of America. J Am Coll Cardiol 2005;46:1144–78.

[3] American Heart Association. Heart disease and stroke statistics—2005 update. Dallas: American Heart Association; 2005.

[4] HCUPnet. Healthcare Cost and Utilization Project. Agency for Healthcare Resource and Quality. Rockville (MD). Available at: http://hcup.ahrq.gov/HCUPnet.asp.

[5] Delgado R, Gregory D, Konstam MA. Temporal changes in US hospitalizations, costs and clinical characteristics of patients with severe acute decompensated heart failure. Eur J Heart Fail 2005;4:80.

[6] Feldman D, Dasta J, McLaughlin T, et al. Comparison of patients with primary vs secondary heart failure from a database of 2.5 million admissions: implications for coding and reimbursement policies. Circulation 2005;111:e345.

[7] Fonarow GC, Corday E. Overview of acutely decompensated congestive heart failure (ADHF): a report from the ADHERE registry. Heart Fail Rev 2004;9:179–85.

[8] Nieminen MS, Harjola VP. Definition and epidemiology of acute heart failure syndromes. Am J Cardiol 2005;96(suppl):5–10.

[9] Adams Jr KF, Fonarow GC, Emerman CL, et al. Characteristics and outcomes of patients hospitalized for heart failure in the United States: rationale, design, and preliminary observations from the first 100,000 cases in the Acute Decompensated Heart Failure National Registry (ADHERE). Am Heart J 2005;149:209–16.

[10] Fonarow GC, Adams Jr KF, Abraham WT, et al. Risk stratification for in-hospital mortality in acutely decompensated heart failure: classification and regression tree analysis. JAMA 2005;293:572–80.

[11] Mann DL. Mechanisms and models in heart failure: a combinatorial approach. Circulation 1999;100:999–1008.

[12] Stevenson LW. Tailored therapy to hemodynamic goals for advanced heart failure. Eur J Heart Fail 1999;1:251–7.

[13] Packer M. The neurohormonal hypothesis: a theory to explain the mechanism of disease progression in heart failure. J Am Coll Cardiol 1992;20:248–54.

[14] Schrier RW, Abraham WT. Hormones and hemodynamics in heart failure. N Engl J Med 1999;341:577–85.

[15] Francis GS, Siegel RM, Goldsmith SR, et al. Acute vasoconstrictor response to intravenous furosemide in patients with chronic congestive heart failure: activation of the neurohumoral axis. Ann Intern Med 1985;103:1–6.

[16] Gottlieb SS, Brater DC, Thomas I, et al. BG9719 (CVT-124), an A1 adenosine receptor antagonist, protects against the decline in renal function observed with diuretic therapy. Circulation 2002;105:1348–53.

[17] Boerrigter G, Burnett Jr JC. Cardiorenal syndrome in decompensated heart failure: prognostic and therapeutic implications. Curr Heart Fail Rep 2004;1:113–20.
[18] Lee SC, Stevens TL, Sandberg SM, et al. The potential of brain natriuretic peptide as a biomarker for New York Heart Association class during the outpatient treatment of heart failure. J Card Fail 2002;8:149–54.
[19] Hirata Y, Matsumoto A, Aoyagi T, et al. Measurement of plasma brain natriuretic peptide level as a guide for cardiac overload. Cardiovasc Res 2001;51:585–91.
[20] Cheng V, Kazanagra R, Garcia A, et al. A rapid bedside test for B-type peptide predicts treatment outcomes in patients admitted for decompensated heart failure: a pilot study. J Am Coll Cardiol 2001;37:386–91.
[21] Hobbs FD, Davis RC, Roalfe AK, et al. Reliability of N-terminal pro-brain natriuretic peptide assay in diagnosis of heart failure: cohort study in representative and high risk community populations. BMJ 2002;324:1498.
[22] Hobbs FD, Davis RC, Roalfe AK, et al. Reliability of N-terminal proBNP assay in diagnosis of left ventricular systolic dysfunction within representative and high risk populations. Heart 2004;90:866–70.
[23] Maisel AS, Koon J, Krishnaswamy P, et al. Utility of B-natriuretic peptide as a rapid, point-of-care test for screening patients undergoing echocardiography to determine left ventricular dysfunction. Am Heart J 2001;141:367–74.
[24] Davis M, Espiner E, Richards G, et al. Plasma brain natriuretic peptide in assessment of acute dyspnoea. Lancet 1994;343:440–4.
[25] McCullough PA, Nowak RM, McCord J, et al. B-type natriuretic peptide and clinical judgment in emergency diagnosis of heart failure: analysis from Breathing Not Properly (BNP) Multinational Study. Circulation 2002;106:416–22.
[26] Lubien E, DeMaria A, Krishnaswamy P, et al. Utility of B-natriuretic peptide in detecting diastolic dysfunction: comparison with Doppler velocity recordings. Circulation 2002;105: 595–601.
[27] Richards AM, Nicholls MG, Yandle TG, et al. Plasma N-terminal pro-brain natriuretic peptide and adrenomedullin: new neurohormonal predictors of left ventricular function and prognosis after myocardial infarction. Circulation 1998;97:1921–9.
[28] Latini R, Masson S, Anand I, et al. The comparative prognostic value of plasma neurohormones at baseline in patients with heart failure enrolled in Val-HeFT. Eur Heart J 2004;25:292–9.
[29] Latini R, Masson S, Anand I, et al. Effects of valsartan on circulating brain natriuretic peptide and norepinephrine in symptomatic chronic heart failure: the Valsartan Heart Failure Trial (Val-HeFT). Circulation 2002;106:2454–8.
[30] Troughton RW, Frampton CM, Yandle TG, et al. Treatment of heart failure guided by plasma aminoterminal brain natriuretic peptide (N-BNP) concentrations. Lancet 2000;355:1126–30.
[31] Domanski MJ, Exner DV, Borkowf CB, et al. Effect of angiotensin converting enzyme inhibition on sudden cardiac death in patients following acute myocardial infarction: a meta-analysis of randomized clinical trials. J Am Coll Cardiol 1999;33:598–604.
[32] Yoshimura M, Mizuno Y, Nakayama M, et al. B-type natriuretic peptide as a marker of the effects of enalapril in patients with heart failure. Am J Med 2002;112:716–20.
[33] Murdoch DR, McDonagh TA, Byrne J, et al. Titration of vasodilator therapy in chronic heart failure according to plasma brain natriuretic peptide concentration: randomized comparison of the hemodynamic and neuroendocrine effects of tailored versus empirical therapy. Am Heart J 1999;138(6 pt 1):1126–32.
[34] Silver MA, Maisel A, Yancy CW, et al. BNP Consensus Panel 2004: a clinical approach for the diagnostic, prognostic, screening, treatment monitoring, and therapeutic roles of natriuretic peptides in cardiovascular diseases. Congest Heart Fail 2004;10(suppl 3):1–30.
[35] Latini R, Masson S, de Angelis N, Anand I. Role of brain natriuretic peptide in the diagnosis and management of heart failure: current concepts. J Card Fail 2002;8:288–99.
[36] Bettencourt PM. Clinical usefulness of B-type natriuretic peptide measurement: present and future perspectives. Heart 2005;91:1489–94.

[37] Binanay C, Califf RM, Hasselblad V, et al. Evaluation study of congestive heart failure and pulmonary artery catheterization effectiveness: the ESCAPE trial. JAMA 2005;294: 1625–33.
[38] Fonarow GC. The treatment targets in acute decompensated heart failure. Rev Cardiovasc Med 2001;2(suppl 2):S7–12.
[39] Cuffe MS, Califf RM, Adams Jr KF, et al. Short-term intravenous milrinone for acute exacerbation of chronic heart failure: a randomized controlled trial. JAMA 2002;287:1541–7.
[40] Leier CV, Webel J, Bush CA. The cardiovascular effects of the continuous infusion of dobutamine in patients with severe cardiac failure. Circulation 1977;56:468–72.
[41] Krell MJ, Kline EM, Bates ER, et al. Intermittent, ambulatory dobutamine infusions in patients with severe congestive heart failure. Am Heart J 1986;112:787–91.
[42] Packer M, Carver JR, Rodeheffer RJ, et al. Effect of oral milrinone on mortality in severe chronic heart failure. The PROMISE Study Research Group. N Engl J Med 1991;325: 1468–75.
[43] Fowler MB. Carvedilol Prospective Randomized Cumulative Survival (COPERNICUS) trial: carvedilol in severe heart failure. Am J Cardiol 2004;93:35B–9B.
[44] Krum H, Roecker EB, Mohacsi P, et al. Effects of initiating carvedilol in patients with severe chronic heart failure: results from the COPERNICUS Study. JAMA 2003;289:712–8.
[45] Brater DC. Diuretic therapy. N Engl J Med 1998;339:387–95.
[46] Brater DC. Diuretic therapy in congestive heart failure. Congest Heart Fail 2000;6:197–201.
[47] Dormans TP, van Meyel JJ, Gerlag PG, et al. Diuretic efficacy of high dose furosemide in severe heart failure: bolus injection versus continuous infusion. J Am Coll Cardiol 1996;28: 376–82.
[48] Pivac N, Rumboldt Z, Sardelic S, et al. Diuretic effects of furosemide infusion versus bolus injection in congestive heart failure. Int J Clin Pharmacol Res 1998;18:121–8.
[49] Aaser E, Gullestad L, Tollofsrud S, et al. Effect of bolus injection versus continuous infusion of furosemide on diuresis and neurohormonal activation in patients with severe congestive heart failure. Scand J Clin Lab Invest 1997;57:361–7.
[50] Lahav M, Regev A, Ra'anani P, Theodor E. Intermittent administration of furosemide vs continuous infusion preceded by a loading dose for congestive heart failure. Chest 1992;102: 725–31.
[51] Gupta S, Neyses L. Diuretic usage in heart failure: a continuing conundrum in 2005. Eur Heart J 2005;26:644–9.
[52] Khot UN, Novaro GM, Popovic ZB, et al. Nitroprusside in critically ill patients with left ventricular dysfunction and aortic stenosis. N Engl J Med 2003;348:1756–63.
[53] Elkayam U, Akhter MW, Singh H, et al. Comparison of effects on left ventricular filling pressure of intravenous nesiritide and high-dose nitroglycerin in patients with decompensated heart failure. Am J Cardiol 2004;93:237–40.
[54] Publication Committee for VMAC Investigators. Intravenous nesiritide vs nitroglycerin for treatment of decompensated congestive heart failure: a randomized controlled trial. JAMA 2002;287:1531–40.
[55] Mills RM, LeJemtel TH, Horton DP, et al. Sustained hemodynamic effects of an infusion of nesiritide (human b-type natriuretic peptide) in heart failure: a randomized, double-blind, placebo-controlled clinical trial. Natrecor Study Group. J Am Coll Cardiol 1999;34:155–62.
[56] Colucci WS, Elkayam U, Horton DP, et al. Intravenous nesiritide, a natriuretic peptide, in the treatment of decompensated congestive heart failure. Nesiritide Study Group. N Engl J Med 2000;343:246–53.
[57] Burger AJ, Elkayam U, Neibaur MT, et al. Comparison of the occurrence of ventricular arrhythmias in patients with acutely decompensated congestive heart failure receiving dobutamine versus nesiritide therapy. Am J Cardiol 2001;88:35–9.
[58] Scios I. Nesiritide (Natrecor) package insert. 2005.
[59] Sackner-Bernstein JD, Skopicki HA, Aaronson KD. Risk of worsening renal function with nesiritide in patients with acutely decompensated heart failure. Circulation 2005;111:1487–91.

[60] Sackner-Bernstein JD, Kowalski M, Fox M, Aaronson K. Short-term risk of death after treatment with nesiritide for decompensated heart failure: a pooled analysis of randomized controlled trials. JAMA 2005;293:1900–5.
[61] Abraham WT, Adams KF, Fonarow GC, et al. In-hospital mortality in patients with acute decompensated heart failure requiring intravenous vasoactive medications: an analysis from the Acute Decompensated Heart Failure National Registry (ADHERE). J Am Coll Cardiol 2005; 46:57–64.
[62] Elkayam U. Nesiritide may diminish the increased acute mortality risk associated with worsening renal function. Circulation 2005;112(suppl):II-675–6.
[63] Felker GM, O'Connor CM. Inotropic therapy for heart failure: an evidence-based approach. Am Heart J 2001;142:393–401.
[64] The Digitalis Investigation Group. The effect of digoxin on mortality and morbidity in patients with heart failure. N Engl J Med 1997;336:525–33.
[65] Elsasser A, Schlepper M, Klovekorn WP, et al. Hibernating myocardium: an incomplete adaptation to ischemia. Circulation 1997;96:2920–31.
[66] Travill CM, Pugh S, Noble MI. The inotropic and hemodynamic effects of intravenous milrinone when reflex adrenergic stimulation is suppressed by beta-adrenergic blockade. Clin Ther 1994;16:783–92.
[67] Goldsmith SR. Current treatments and novel pharmacologic treatments for hyponatremia in congestive heart failure. Am J Cardiol 2005;95:14B–23B.
[68] Naitoh M, Risvanis J, Balding LC, et al. Neurohormonal antagonism in heart failure; beneficial effects of vasopressin V(1a) and V(2) receptor blockade and ACE inhibition. Cardiovasc Res 2002;54:51–7.
[69] Yatsu T, Tomura Y, Tahara A, et al. Pharmacological profile of YM087, a novel nonpeptide dual vasopressin V1A and V2 receptor antagonist, in dogs. Eur J Pharmacol 1997;321:225–30.
[70] Gheorghiade M, Gattis WA, O'Connor CM, et al. Effects of tolvaptan, a vasopressin antagonist, in patients hospitalized with worsening heart failure: a randomized controlled trial. JAMA 2004;291:1963–71.
[71] Udelson JE, Smith WB, Hendrix GH, et al. Acute hemodynamic effects of conivaptan, a dual V(1A) and V(2) vasopressin receptor antagonist, in patients with advanced heart failure. Circulation 2001;104:2417–23.
[72] Ng TM. Levosimendan, a new calcium-sensitizing inotrope for heart failure. Pharmacotherapy 2004;24:1366–84.
[73] Mebazaa A, Erhardt L. Levosimendan: a new dual-action drug in the treatment of acute heart failure. Int J Clin Pract 2003;57:410–6.
[74] Moiseyev VS, Poder P, Andrejevs N, et al. Safety and efficacy of a novel calcium sensitizer, levosimendan, in patients with left ventricular failure due to an acute myocardial infarction: a randomized, placebo-controlled, double-blind study (RUSSLAN). Eur Heart J 2002;23: 1422–32.
[75] Ng TM, Akhter MW. Levosimendan: dual mechanisms for acute heart failure and beyond? Min Cardioangiol 2005;53:565–84.
[76] Follath F, Cleland JG, Just H, et al. Efficacy and safety of intravenous levosimendan compared with dobutamine in severe low-output heart failure (the LIDO study): a randomised double-blind trial. Lancet 2002;360:196–202.
[77] Coletta AP, Cleland JG, Freemantle N, Clark AL. Clinical trials update from the European Society of Cardiology Heart Failure meeting: SHAPE, BRING-UP 2 VAS, COLA II, FOSIDIAL, BETACAR, CASINO and meta-analysis of cardiac resynchronisation therapy. Eur J Heart Fail 2004;6:673–6.
[78] Crozier IG, Richards AM, Nicholls MG, et al. Atrial natriuretic factor in human pathophysiology. Clin Exp Pharmacol Physiol 1988;15:173–83.
[79] Ishikawa C, Tsutamoto T, Wada A, et al. Inhibition of aldosterone and endothelin-1 by carperitide was attenuated with more than 1 week of infusion in patients with congestive heart failure. J Cardiovasc Pharmacol 2005;46:513–8.

[80] Hummel M, Kuhn M, Bub A, et al. Urodilatin, a new therapy to prevent kidney failure after heart transplantation. J Heart Lung Transplant 1993;12:209–17.
[81] Elsner D, Muders F, Muntze A, et al. Efficacy of prolonged infusion of urodilatin [ANP-(95–126)] in patients with congestive heart failure. Am Heart J 1995;129:766–73.
[82] Forssmann W, Meyer M, Forssmann K. The renal urodilatin system: clinical implications. Cardiovasc Res 2001;51:450–62.
[83] Suwa M, Seino Y, Nomachi Y, et al. Multicenter prospective investigation on efficacy and safety of carperitide for acute heart failure in the 'real world' of therapy. Circ J 2005;69:283–90.
[84] Kikuchi M, Nakamura M, Suzuki T, et al. Usefulness of carperitide for the treatment of refractory heart failure due to severe acute myocardial infarction. Jpn Heart J 2001;42:271–80.
[85] Gottlieb SS, Skettino SL, Wolff A, et al. Effects of BG9719 (CVT-124), an A1-adenosine receptor antagonist, and furosemide on glomerular filtration rate and natriuresis in patients with congestive heart failure. J Am Coll Cardiol 2000;35:56–9.
[86] Gottlieb SS. Renal effects of adenosine A1-receptor antagonists in congestive heart failure. Drugs 2001;61:1387–93.
[87] Grapsa E, Alexopoulos GP, Margari Z, et al. Ultrafiltration in the treatment of severe congestive heart failure. Int Urol Nephrol 2004;36:269–72.
[88] Sharma A, Hermann DD, Mehta RL. Clinical benefit and approach of ultrafiltration in acute heart failure. Cardiology 2001;96:144–54.
[89] Peacock WF. Clinical and economic impact of nesiritide. Am J Health Syst Pharm 2003;60(suppl):S21–6.
[90] Long J, Proach J. Incidence and potential economic impact of hyponatremia in hospitalized patients. Pharmacotherapy 2005;25:1476.
[91] Yamani MH, Haji SA, Starling RC, et al. Comparison of dobutamine-based and milrinone-based therapy for advanced decompensated congestive heart failure: hemodynamic efficacy, clinical outcome, and economic impact. Am Heart J 2001;142:998–1002.
[92] Cleland JG, Takala A, Apajasalo M, et al. Intravenous levosimendan treatment is cost-effective compared with dobutamine in severe low-output heart failure: an analysis based on the international LIDO trial. Eur J Heart Fail 2003;5:101–8.
[93] de Lissovoy G, Stier DM, Ciesla G, et al. Economic implications of nesiritide versus dobutamine in the treatment of patients with acutely decompensated congestive heart failure. Am J Cardiol 2003;92:631–3.
[94] Gerhard T, Zineh I, Winterstein A, Hartzema A. Pharmacoeconomic modeling of nesiritide versus dobutamine for decompensated heart failure. Pharmacotherapy 2006;26:34–43.
[95] Lenz TL, Foral PA, Malesker MA, et al. Impact of nesiritide on health care resource utilization and complications in patients with decompensated heart failure. Pharmacotherapy 2004;24:1137–46.
[96] Blackburn J, DiDomenico RJ, Hilleman DE, et al. Early therapy with nesiritide in hospitalized patients with acute decompensated heart failure associated with reduced costs: a Markov analysis. J Card Fail 2005;11:S178.
[97] Peacock WFT, Holland R, Gyarmathy R, et al. Observation unit treatment of heart failure with nesiritide: results from the proaction trial. J Emerg Med 2005;29:243–52.
[98] DiDomenico RJ, Park HY, Southworth MR, et al. Guidelines for acute decompensated heart failure treatment. Ann Pharmacother 2004;38:649–60.
[99] Eyrich HM, DiDomenico RJ, Fontana D, et al. Treatment guidelines for acute decompensated heart failure associated with improved outcomes. Pharmacotherapy 2005;25:1435.

ELSEVIER
SAUNDERS

Crit Care Clin 22 (2006) 221–243

CRITICAL
CARE
CLINICS

Effect of Vasoactive Therapy on Cerebral Circulation

Denise H. Rhoney, PharmD*, Xi Liu-DeRyke, PharmD

Department of Pharmacy Practice, Eugene Applebaum College of Pharmacy and Health Sciences, Wayne State University, 259 Mack Avenue, Detroit, MI 48201, USA

The incidence of new and recurrent stroke is approximately 700,000 annually in the United States, resulting in 162,672 deaths and $56.8 billion in health care expenditures, which makes stroke a principal cause of disability and an economic burden on society [1]. Acute ischemic stroke (AIS) accounts for more than 80% of all stroke, and hemorrhagic stroke, including intracerebral hemorrhage (ICH) and subarachnoid hemorrhage, makes up the remaining 20%. Malignant hypertension is a significant risk factor and major complication of all acute strokes. Approximately two thirds of the patients who have a first stroke have a history of hypertension [1]. In addition, acute hypertension is observed in 80% of patients after a stroke, irrespective of a previous history of hypertension. This initial increase in the blood pressure is believed to be a protective mechanism by the brain for maintaining cerebral perfusion pressure (CPP). A persistent increase in blood pressure can lead to hemorrhagic transformation, rebleeding, or brain edema, however, which may result in secondary stroke or further neurologic damage.

Managing blood pressure during the acute phase of a stroke is a challenge. In the International Stroke Trial (IST), high and low blood pressures were independent prognostic factors for poor outcomes [2]. This indicates that a delicate balance of blood pressure management is vital in ensuring a successful outcome in patients with brain injury. Additionally, a spontaneous decrease in blood pressure without receiving treatment was documented a few days after stroke onset [3,4]. This observation further complicates the decision of whether to treat hypertension acutely in patients with stroke. There is a lack of consensus on

D.H. Rhoney has received an unrestricted educational grant from ESP Pharma.

* Corresponding author.

E-mail address: drhoney@wayne.edu (D.H. Rhoney).

doi:10.1016/j.ccc.2006.02.009 ***criticalcare.theclinics.com***

whether to treat the transient elevation in blood pressure after stroke and on how aggressive blood pressure should be lowered in AIS and primary ICH. The general belief is that acute hypertension should be treated so as to avoid secondary neuronal damage; however, adequate perfusion to the brain must also be maintained. The management of acute hypertension after stroke varies greatly throughout the world among neurologists and neurosurgeons despite existing guidelines. Therefore, understanding cerebral physiology and the pharmacokinetic and pharmacodynamic properties of antihypertensive agents is vital in guiding therapeutic decisions in these patients.

Cerebrovascular physiology

The pathophysiology of stroke is a multifaceted process involving cellular and metabolic abnormalities (ion imbalance, inflammation, and cell death), endothelial damage, and vascular changes. The focus of this review is on understanding the vascular changes that occur after stroke and how this aids in decision making.

Normal physiology

When considering patients with acute neurologic disease, maintenance of cerebral blood flow (CBF) is the key goal. In healthy individuals, the brain has little capacity to store oxygen; therefore, it is imperative to maintain a relatively constant CBF to ensure adequate cerebral oxygen supply for the metabolic requirement. To understand the relation among mean arterial pressure (MAP), intracranial pressure (ICP), CBF, and CPP, it is important to have a thorough knowledge of the normal cerebral physiology. CBF is regulated through CPP and cerebral vascular resistance (CVR), and these relations are expressed mathematically as follows:

$$CPP = MAP - ICP$$

$$CBF = CPP/CVR$$

The body protects the brain by a hemostatic mechanism known as cerebral autoregulation. Autoregulation can be defined as the inherent ability of arteries to vasodilate (decrease in CVR) or vasoconstrict (increase in CVR) in response to changing perfusion pressure to maintain a relatively stable CBF (Fig. 1). CPP generally approximates MAP when the brain is free of trauma or injury. Under normal circumstances, the brain is able to maintain a constant CBF of approximately 50 mL per 100 g/min over a wide range of MAP ranging from approximately 60 to 150 mm Hg. The brain resides within a rigid cranial vault that is protected by the skull. Within this incompressible compartment, brain tissue (80%), cerebral spinal fluid (10%), and blood (10%) are in a state of equilibrium.

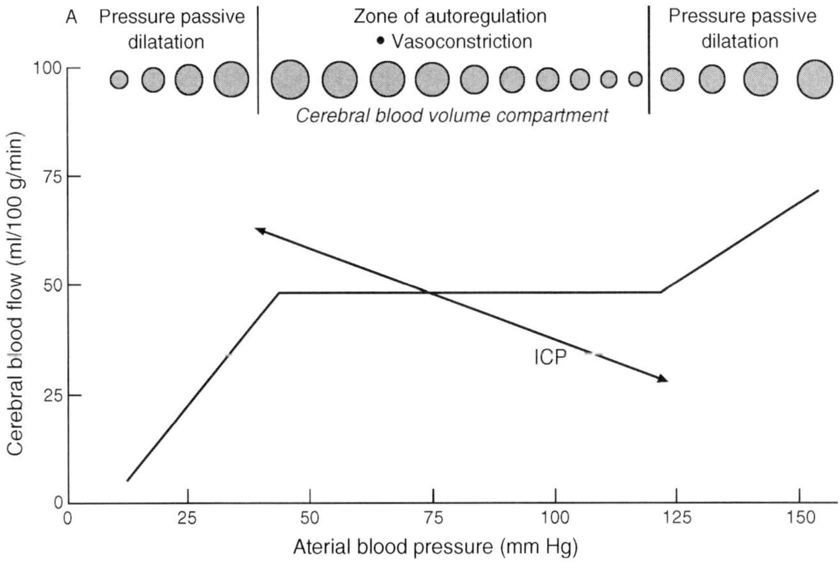

Fig. 1. Normal cerebral autoregulation curve. With normal cerebral physiology, the brain maintains constant CBF under a wide range of MAPs (range: 60–150 mm Hg). When MAP falls below or exceeds the limits of autoregulation, CBF becomes pressure dependent. (*From* Lang EW. Cerebral vasomotor reactivity testing in head injury: the link between pressure and flow. J Neurol Neurosurg Psychiatry 2003;74(8):1054; with permission.)

Any change in one component of the brain needs to be compensated for by a decrease in one or more of the other components. When the intracranial vault volume is disturbed, ICP increases, which causes a reduction in CPP. The reduction in CPP can decrease CBF when autoregulation is disrupted (see Fig. 1).

After a decrease in CBF, the body initially compensates by increasing the oxygen extraction fraction from the blood. Cerebral ischemia eventually occurs when the pressure remains low or below the lower limit of autoregulation, however. Conversely, cerebral vessels constrict as MAP rises and the vascular endothelial cells become stretched. Eventually, the cerebral vessels can no longer constrict effectively against the high perfusion pressure, and autoregulation fails, leading to cerebral edema or hemorrhage. In patients with chronic hypertension, the autoregulatory curve is shifted to the right toward higher pressures. Therefore, lowering the blood pressure to a "normal range" in patients with poorly controlled chronic hypertension may accelerate end-organ damage because of the lack of oxygen perfusion to the tissues. In addition, patients with neurologic injury (eg, stroke) may have impaired autoregulation, and CBF becomes pressure dependent [5]. In this scenario, a small change in blood pressure can have a drastic impact on CBF, and thus can affect oxygen supply to the brain.

Overall, the debate for managing blood pressure during the acute phase of stroke centers on two theories. First, hypertension is a risk factor for developing stroke, and elevated blood pressure during the acute phase can lead to neurologic deterioration by promoting cerebral edema and hemorrhage. Second, actively lowering blood pressure during the acute phase may adversely affect cerebral perfusion, resulting in further stroke and worsening neurologic outcome. It is essential to understand the evidence supporting or negating these theories in AIS and ICH to assess when it is appropriate to initiate acute antihypertensive therapy.

Significance of hypertension in acute ischemic stroke

Before considering acute blood pressure management in AIS, understanding the concept of the penumbra is crucial (Fig. 2). Ischemic stroke results from occlusion of cerebral vessels, which leads to a decrease in blood flow and deprivation of oxygen supply to the brain. The normal CBF is approximately 50 mL per 100 g/min. In the focal region with infarction, CBF is generally diminished (less than 10 mL per 100 g/min). This hypoperfusion results in permanent neuronal damage, and this part of the tissue is known as the ischemic core. The ischemic penumbra is the area immediately surrounding the ischemic core, where CBF is decreased (10–20 mL per 100 g/min), but the tissue can be salvageable if reperfusion is established. This concept was first proposed by Astrup and colleagues [6] in 1981 and has since been validated with imaging studies using positron emission tomography, diffusion-weighted imaging, and MRI. Within the penumbra, blood flow is sufficient to maintain cellular viability acutely but not sufficient for normal cellular function. It is therefore essential to provide adequate perfusion to this area promptly so as to limit the extension of the ischemic core.

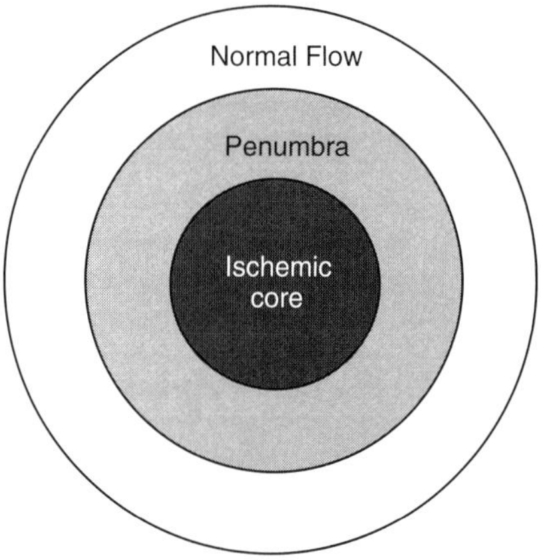

Fig. 2. Relation between ischemic core, penumbra, and normal cells after ischemic stroke. After AIS, CBF diminishes (<10 mL per 100 g/min) within a focal region and immediate cell death occurs, resulting in an ischemic core. The surrounding tissue, called the penumbra, is supplied by decreased CBF (10–20 mL per 100 g/min); however, cell death can be avoided if reperfusion to the area is established. Within unaffected cerebral tissues, CBF is approximately 50 mL per 100 g/min.

The goal of keeping adequate perfusion and oxygenation to the brain lays the foundation for the argument not to lower blood pressure acutely after stroke. Eames and coworkers [7] found a loss of integrity of autoregulation in patients with AIS after they were matched with individuals without stroke for age, gender, and MAP. The results confirmed the theory that neurologic injury leads to impairment of cerebral autoregulation, and CBF becomes pressure dependent. Aggressive lowering of the blood pressure thus results in a reduction in CBF and compromises the perfusion and oxygenation to the brain. Okumura and colleagues [8] sought to delineate the correlation between admission blood pressure and mortality and how the relations may differ in stroke types in a large population. A total of 2101 patients, 1004 with AIS and 1097 with primary ICH, were enrolled and eligible for the analysis. In patients with ischemic stroke, systolic blood pressure (SBP; <130 or >210 mm Hg) and diastolic blood pressure (DBP; <70 or >110 mm Hg) were associated with a 1.6- to 3.5-fold risk of mortality in 30 days after stroke. This finding confirmed the U-shaped relation of blood pressure and outcomes in patients with ischemic stroke. In addition, the study demonstrated that patients with a history of hypertension needed a higher blood pressure to survive compared with those without such a history. This finding supported the theory of the autoregulation curve shifted toward the right in patients with chronic uncontrolled hypertension, in which case, overaggressive lowering of blood pressure may adversely affect the cerebral perfusion. In fact, this evidence may suggest the need to elevate blood pressure with vasopressor agents in an effort to increase CPP and improve CBF. Induced hypertension has not become a common practice outside the setting of severe hypotension and would require further clinical study, although there are recent reports evaluating this treatment modality [9,10].

Meanwhile, a meta-analysis [11] examined the relation between the admission blood pressure and clinical outcomes in more than 10,000 patients, including patients with AIS and ICH. Elevated SBP (150–200 mm Hg), MAP (140–145 mm Hg), and DBP (90–115 mm Hg) were associated with early recurrence, increased disability, and death, irrespective of stroke type. In addition, several observational studies have shown that elevated blood pressure after ischemic infarct leads to brain edema and hemorrhagic transformation, suggesting that there may be a scientific base for acutely lowering blood pressure after stroke.

Because of the conflicting facts and limited evidence, blood pressure management in AIS remains controversial. Acknowledging limitations in the currently published literature, the Stroke Council of the American Stroke Association made the following recommendation regarding blood pressure management in patients with AIS [12,13]. In patients who are not eligible for thrombolytic therapy, blood pressure is treated only when the SBP is greater than 220 mm Hg or the DBP is greater than 140 mmHg, and the goal is to lower the blood pressure by 10% to 15% from baseline. The threshold of treatment is lower in patients who are eligible for thrombolytic therapy. Treatment is initiated when the SBP is greater than 185 mm Hg or the DBP is greater than 110 mm Hg, and the goal is to maintain the blood pressure below the treatment threshold [12,13].

Significance of hypertension in primary intracerebral hemorrhage

Patients with primary ICH admitted to the hospital were found to have significantly higher blood pressure compared with patients with AIS [8,11,14]. Okumura and colleagues [8] demonstrated a U-shaped relation between the admission DBP and mortality in patients with primary ICH, whereas the SBP seemed to have a J-shaped relation. A SBP greater than 190 mm Hg was associated with a twofold risk of death, and the risk increased to fourfold when the SBP was greater than 230 mm Hg. This relationship between elevated blood pressure on hospital admission and poor clinical outcomes was confirmed by several other studies [15–17]. There also seems to be a correlation between high blood pressure and hematoma expansion, which is an independent factor for further neurologic deterioration and poor clinical outcome. The causative relationship between high blood pressure and hematoma expansion after spontaneous ICH remains debatable. Ohwaki and coworkers [18] examined the relation between blood pressure and hematoma expansion in 76 patients with ICH. Approximately 20% of patients experienced hematoma enlargement in which an elevated SBP ($\geq$160 mm Hg) was an independent factor for enlargement (odds ratio [OR] = 1.041, 95% confidence interval [CI], 1.01–1.074). Conversely, Kazui and colleagues [16] found that high SBP was a risk factor for hematoma expansion only in poorly controlled diabetes. Fujii and coworkers [19] identified five independent risk factors for hematoma expansion; however, increased blood pressure was not found to be a significant predictor. Whether elevated blood pressure is the cause of hematoma expansion or vice versa is yet to be delineated.

Because of the discovery of the penumbra in AIS, concern remains regarding the potential adverse effects of blood pressure lowering during the acute phase of ICH. In theory, possible ischemic events in the brain tissue surrounding the hematoma may be associated with a rapid decrease in blood pressure. Therefore, leaving the blood pressure alone after ICH may prevent hypoperfusion and a subsequent ischemic event. The evidence for the penumbra area in ICH is weak, however. In an experimental ICH model, Qureshi and colleagues [20] examined the effect of MAP reduction on the regional cerebral blood flow (rCBF) and whether ischemia existed around the periclot region. Labetalol was administered 90 minutes after the introduction of ICH in dogs to keep MAP greater than 65 mm Hg. Compared with control animals (surgery only), no difference in rCBF was detected in any zone around the injury. More importantly, an increase in ICP and MAP was observed after the induction of ICH. A significant reduction in MAP was noted after administering labetalol; however, no significant change in ICP and CPP was noted. A decrease in CVR was observed, indicating that autoregulation was intact when the blood pressure was lowered in a controlled fashion, and there was no evidence of periclot ischemia in the acute phase of ICH. Similar findings were reported in clinical studies (Table 1) [21–26]. In these studies, a reduction in the global CBF was observed; however, it is suggested that the hypoperfusion was indicative of a

Table 1
Autoregulation and ischemic penumbra in primary intracerebral hemorrhage

Study	Design	Significant findings
Kuwata et al [21] (1995)	68 ICH patients	No dysautoregulation was observed
	Antihypertensive agent: trimethaphan or diltiazem	Acute phase: no effect on MAP with BP reduction <20%
Carhuapoma et al [22] (2000)	9 ICH patients	Vasogenic edema was observed around the hematoma
	DW MRI and proton MR spectroscopic imaging	No evidence of ischemia adjacent to the hematoma
	Time to imaging: mean 3.4 days	
Kidwell et al [23] (2001)	12 ICH patients	6 patients underwent PWI: no focal ischemia around the hematoma
	DWI and PWI	5 of 6 patients had ipsilateral hypoperfusion
	Time to imaging: <6 hours	
Zazulia AR et al [24] (2001)	19 ICH patients	Global decrease in CBF, $CMRO_2$, and OEF in periclot region compared with contralateral region
	PET: 5–22 hours after onset	No ischemia during the hyperacute stage
Powers et al [25] (2001)	14 ICH patients	No significant change in global CBF and rCBF after BP reduction
	PET: 6–22 hours	No correlation between reduction in MAP and global CBF or rCBF
	Antihypertensive agent: nicardipine or labetalol	Autoregulation remained intact when MAP lowered by 10%–22%
	Lower MAP by 15%	
Schellinger PD et al [26] (2003)	32 ICH patients	Perihematoma hypoperfusion indicating a reduced metabolic demand
	DWI and PWI	No signs of salvageable penumbra
	Time to imaging: <6 hours	

Abbreviations: BP blood pressure; CBF, cerebral blood flow; $CMRO_2$, cerebral metabolic rate of oxygen consumption; DWI, diffusion-weighted imaging; DW MRI, diffusion-weighted magnetic resonance imaging; ICH, intracerebral hemorrhage; MAP, mean arterial pressure; OEF, oxygen extraction fraction; PET, positron emission tomography; PWI, perfusion-weighted imaging; rCBF, regional cerebral blood flow.

reduction in cerebral metabolism during the hyperacute stage of ICH rather than an ischemic event.

Because of the lack of convincing evidence of a penumbra area in acute primary ICH and the potential relation to hematoma growth in the presence of elevated blood pressure, blood pressure reduction during the acute phase of primary ICH is likely to be safe. Moreover, autoregulation seems to be preserved with controlled blood pressure lowering [21,25]. Powers and coworkers [25] investigated the effect of blood pressure lowering on autoregulation of CBF in patients with small to medium ICH (1–45 mL). They found that autoregulation of CBF was not adversely effected when the lower MAP limit was 110 mm Hg or a 20% or less reduction from the baseline. Nevertheless, larger trials are needed to (1) identify whether a penumbra area is present in patients with a large hematoma volume (>45 mL), (2) identify the safest lower limit for lowering blood pressure, and (3) identify how fast the blood pressure should be lowered. Currently, a National Institutes of Health (NIH)–funded study (NCT00226096) expecting to enroll 4000 patients is underway to establish the effect of intensive blood pressure lowering to different thresholds in acute ICH on morbidity and mortality [27].

Pharmacotherapy

Thus far, evidence indicates that acute blood pressure management may be beneficial in stroke to prevent neurologic deterioration; however, this needs to be done in a controlled fashion, and moderation of blood pressure lowering is important for preserving cerebral perfusion. Therefore, an ideal vasoactive agent should have minimum cerebral effects (ie, CBF, ICP), a predictable dose response (avoidance of precipitous drops in blood pressure that can lead to hypoperfusion and end-organ damage), and rapid onset and offset of action. In addition, because many patients have comorbidities, consideration should be given to the risk of drug interactions and likelihood of exacerbating comorbid conditions. To help clinicians make a rational choice as to whether blood pressure is deemed as needing treatment, we now review the systemic and cerebral effects of commonly used intravenous antihypertensive agents and their therapeutic application in patients with stroke. Table 2 summarizes the physiologic and cerebrovascular effects of selected intravenous antihypertensive agents.

Sodium nitroprusside

Cardiovascular effect

Nitroprusside is the most widely used parenteral agent for the management of hypertensive crisis, attributed to its fast onset and short duration of action. It is normally given as an intravenous infusion with immediate onset of action and effects lasting 2 to 3 minutes after termination in relatively healthy individuals [28]. Nitroprusside is a potent venous and arterial vasodilator, which results

Table 2
Systemic and cerebral physiologic effects of antihypertensive agents

	Heart rate	Cardiac output	Mean arterial pressure	Intracerebral pressure	Cerebral perfusion pressure	Cerebral blood flow
Nitroprusside	↑	↑ ↓	↓	↑	↓?	↑ ↓↔
Nitroglycerin	↑	↓	↓	↑	↓?	↓?
Esmolol	↓	↑	↓	?	↓?	↓?
Labetalol	↓	↑	↓	↔?	↓?	↔?
Nicardipine	↔	↑	↓	↔	↓↔	↑↔
Enalaprilat	↔	↑↔	↓	?	↓?	↑↔
Hydralazine	↑	↑ ↓	↓	↑	↓	↑↔
Fenoldopam	↑↔	↑	↓	↑?	↓?	↓?

Abbreviations: ↑ , increase; ↓, decrease; ↔, no change; ?, unknown.

in a reduction in vascular resistance and, consequently, a reduction in preload and afterload. These properties make nitroprusside useful in treating hypertensive patients with underlying pulmonary edema or congestive heart failure. Meanwhile, studies suggest that nitroprusside can cause "coronary steal" through redistribution of blood flow away from the heart, resulting in reduced coronary perfusion pressure [29–31]. Other disadvantages of nitroprusside include tachyphylaxis and the need for a special delivery system because of its photosensitivity.

One of the major drawbacks of nitroprusside is the accumulation of toxic metabolites, which has been associated with high doses, prolonged use, and end-organ dysfunction. Nitroprusside contains 44% cyanide by weight, which is released by smooth muscles in a dose-dependent manner. Cyanide toxicity results from binding of cyanide to the heme molecule of mitochondrial cytochrome oxidase, resulting in cellular hypoxia. In healthy individuals, toxic levels of cyanide can be expected in 500 minutes in an 80-kg adult receiving an infusion at a rate of 2 μg/kg/min [32]. Monitoring for cyanide toxicity is often difficult, because the utility of cyanide concentrations is questionable; thus, monitoring is left to clinical evaluation [33]. Tachyphylaxis is often thought to be an indication of impending toxicity. In addition, a direct relation between lactic acidosis and serum cyanide concentrations exists [34]. Cyanide is further metabolized by the liver to thiocyanate and excreted through the kidney. Therefore, thiocyanate toxicity is particularly problematic in patients with renal impairment, and it can accumulate as soon as 3 days after an infusion is started. Cyanide and thiocyanate toxicities can be difficult to diagnose, because symptoms (mostly of the central nervous system [CNS]) are similar to those seen with CNS injury. Thus, the possibility of cyanide or thiocyanate toxicity demands attention in all patients receiving nitroprusside infusion, because toxicity can occur rapidly, be fatal, and is difficult to identify in these patients.

Cerebrovascular effect

The theoretic concern of using nitroprusside in patients with brain injury is that nitroprusside dilates cerebral vessels, unselectively resulting in an increase in CBF and, consequently, ICP. Case reports and studies [35–37] have demonstrated a direct correlation between increased ICP and nitroprusside infusion. Cottrell and colleagues [35] demonstrated a linear relation between ICP and the degree of blood pressure reduction in 10 patients with intracranial mass lesions. The potential mechanism of increased ICP in these patients is that the intracranial volume was disturbed because of the mass effect (ie, tumor, hematoma) and that ICP increases as a result of administering an agent that can increase cerebral blood volume. Concurrently, a significant decrease in CPP was observed during nitroprusside infusion.

Nitroprusside and its effect on CBF are less clear because of mixed results published in the literature. Data supporting that nitroprusside does not adversely affect CBF were reported in several studies [38–41]. In one report [38], nine patients received nitroprusside infusion under general anesthesia. CBF, cerebral metabolic rate of oxygen consumption ($CMRO_2$), CVR, and CPP were collected before, during, and after the infusion. A reduction in CVR and CPP was observed, along with a reduction in blood pressure. Changes in CBF and $CMRO_2$ were insignificant throughout the study, however. In two patients who experienced a significant increase in CBF during the infusion, no major impact on cerebral oxygen uptake was observed. There were also data indicating that nitroprusside-induced hypotension resulted in an increase in CBF [35,42,43]; yet, other studies reported that the use of nitroprusside was associated with a decrease in CBF [44–47].

Reasons for such variability in the cerebral response to nitroprusside are not easily determined; however, many of these studies were conducted in the operating suite. Differences in anesthetic technique (anesthetic agents are known to affect CBF, $CMRO_2$, ICP, CVR, and CPP), baseline comorbidities among patients, type of neurologic injury, and the integrity of the autoregulatory system may all contribute to such variation. Patients with impaired autoregulation (eg, patients with stroke) are especially susceptible to the sudden change in blood pressure. In these patients, a small reduction in blood pressure induced by nitroprusside may result in significant changes in CBF and an increased ICP. Hypo- or hyperperfusion may ensue and lead to further brain injury.

Therapeutic implications

In patients with preexisting impairment of cerebrovascular autoregulation, a sudden variation in MAP induced by nitroprusside may exceed the capacity of the cerebral circulation to autoregulate its flow. In addition, patients with an intracranial mass (eg, hematoma) have an increased intracranial volume. This increased volume causes an increase in ICP, and an abrupt drop in MAP can decrease cerebral perfusion. Therefore, even though nitroprusside is still one of the first-line agents recommended by stroke guidelines for acute hypertension management, caution should be exercised; its use requires careful monitoring of CBF, CPP, and ICP, especially in patients who may have altered intracranial compliance or disturbances in autoregulation.

Nitroglycerin

Cardiovascular effect

Nitroglycerin is an organic nitrate and exhibits different pharmacologic effects and toxicity profiles than nitroprusside. At lower doses, nitroglycerin is a potent venodilator, causing a reduction in preload, and has little effect on arteriolar resistance and systemic arterial pressure. At higher doses, nitroglycerin further dilates venous smooth muscles as well as arterioles, which reduces arterial blood pressure and activates sympathetic reflexes (compensatory mechanism). When the compensatory mechanism fails under the prolonged venous pooling, serious systemic hypotension and intravascular hypovolemia occur. Because nitroglycerin dilates primarily capacitance and postcapillary resistance vessels, which account for approximately 80% of regional blood volume and 15% of pressure drop, it is not an effective antihypertensive agent and its hypotensive effect is less predictable [30,48]. Nitroglycerin, however, is an effective antianginal agent because of its ability to increase the collateral blood supply to the heart and reduce oxygen consumption. The seventh report from the Joint National Committee recommends nitroglycerin for hypertensive patients with acute coronary syndromes, such as myocardial infarction [26]. Nitroglycerin also causes arteriolar dilation in the face and neck irrespective of dose, resulting in flushing and severe headache. Tolerance is likely to develop with continuous use, which results in attenuation of pharmacologic effects and generally is resolved with a nitrate-free interval.

Cerebrovascular effect

Although the debate about using nitroprusside in patients with cerebrovascular diseases continues, some have suggested using nitroglycerin as an alternative based on limited data in cerebral vasospasm [49]. Headaches induced by nitroglycerin suggest its dilatory effect on cerebral vessels, which introduces similar concerns as with nitroprusside. Nitroglycerin is a more potent venodilator than nitroprusside and has a greater effect on capacitance and resistance vessels; therefore, it is more likely to increase CBF and cerebral volume. The net effect of changes in cerebrovasculature is an elevation in ICP, which is more prominent in patients with altered intracranial compliance. Studies examining the cerebral effects of nitroglycerin are scarce. An increase in ICP after the initiation of nitroglycerin has been described in a few experimental and human reports, particularly in patients with compromised autoregulation [50]. Gagnon and coworkers [51] reported their experience with nitroglycerin in a 67-year-old man with a brain tumor. Nitroglycerin was administered twice to this patient, whose ICP had increased from 18 to 40 mm Hg and from 20 to 48 mm Hg, respectively. Both incidences occurred within 2.5 minutes of nitroglycerin infusion. Similarly, Ohar and colleagues [52] observed nitroglycerin-induced intracranial hypertension in a 59-year-old woman with systemic hypertension and pulmonary hypertension. This patient exhibited clinical symptoms of increased ICP, including headache, vomiting, and progressive impaired consciousness. A lumbar puncture was performed with an opening pressure of 210 mm H_2O. This patient regained consciousness, and her neurologic deficits were subsequently resolved after the cession of nitroglycerin infusion.

Therapeutic implications

In neurologic patients with normal intracranial pathologic findings, short-term use of nitroglycerin may be tolerated with transient increases in ICP. In patients with suspected or documented elevated ICP (cerebral tumors or hematoma), perfusion in the brain is particularly susceptible to any changes in blood pressure; therefore, great caution should be exercised when using nitroglycerin in patients with compromised intracranial compliance. Patients with concomitant myocardial infarction may be candidates for nitroglycerin; however, the risk versus benefit should be weighted before administering this agent. In addition, nitroglycerin paste may not be an optimal antihypertensive agent in patients with stroke because it is not easy to titrate and may have residual effects.

β-receptor antagonists

Cardiovascular effect

Esmolol and labetalol are the two most commonly used parenteral β-adrenergic antagonists. Esmolol is a β_1-selective antagonist with a rapid onset of action and short half-life. It is metabolized by blood esterases; therefore, the clearance of the drug is independent of liver and renal function. Esmolol is primarily used for supraventricular tachycardia as well as for intraoperative or postoperative hypertension. The major concern with this medication is that severe bradycardia can develop before lowering of blood pressure is observed; therefore, it is not routinely used for the treatment of a hypertensive crisis.

Unlike esmolol or other pure β-adrenergic antagonists, labetalol is a mixed α_1-, β_1-, and β_2-antagonist. Its beta-blockade activity is approximately seven times that of alpha-blockade after intravenous administration. Because labetalol has an effect on both adrenergic receptors, it possesses less of an effect on heart rate and cardiac output compared with other beta-blockers. The onset of action of labetalol is approximately 5 minutes. The duration of action is between 3 and 6 hours, which makes it difficult to titrate as a continuous infusion. Similar to other β-antagonists, labetalol should be avoided in patients with first-degree heart block, severe bradycardia, and asthma.

Cerebrovascular effect

The cerebrovascular effect of labetalol is primarily drawn from healthy volunteers and chronic hypertensive patients. In 1979, Griffith and coworkers [53] reported the effects of chronic use of four beta-blockers (labetalol, metoprolol, oxprenolol, and sotalol) on blood pressure and CBF. A universal reduction in blood pressure was observed as expected; however, no change in CBF was observed before or after treatment. These authors concluded that beta-blockers have little impact on cerebral circulation in the chronic setting but that more research was warranted because their effects may vary during acute administration. Another study [54] conducted in eight healthy normotensive volunteers examined the effects of labetalol on blood pressure, global CBF and rCBF, $CMRO_2$, and cerebral autoregulation. Similar to previous findings, no change in global CBF and rCBF or $CMRO_2$ was detected. The autoregulatory curve was successfully plotted in all participants, and there was no difference in MAP before and after drug infusion. Results from this study indicated that labetalol has little effect on cerebral circulation in the normal brain.

Despite a lack of data on cerebrovascular effects in patients with neurologic injuries, labetalol has been widely used for blood pressure management in these patients. Patel and colleagues [55] examined the efficacy (blood pressure response) of labetalol in patients with hemorrhagic stroke. A moderate lowering in blood pressure (3%–26%) was observed with doses ranging from 5 to 25 mg.

In addition, no worsening of neurologic deficits occurred after administration of the drug. Powers and coworkers [26] further examined the effect of systemic blood pressure lowering on CBF using nicardipine or labetalol in patients with ICH within 6 to 22 hours after onset. Fourteen patients were included in the study (7 were given nicardipine and 7 were given labetalol); MAP and global and periclot CBF were measured and compared with the patients' own baseline. The major conclusions were that a reduction in MAP, up to 20% from baseline, seemed to be safe and that nicardipine and labetalol preserved autoregulation of CBF in patients with ICH.

Therapeutic implication

On the basis of available data, labetalol seems to be a suitable antihypertensive agent in patients with neurologic injuries because it did not demonstrate any negative impact on CBF or autoregulation in healthy patients and patients with ICH. Larger studies are needed to delineate the impact of labetalol on cerebral circulation when autoregulation is impaired. A retrospective study [56] noted that frequent boluses of labetalol were needed to achieve goal blood pressure, requiring more nursing time and frequent monitoring. Further investigation evaluating the effective labetalol dose and time to blood pressure response may have an economic impact on clinical practice.

Calcium channel antagonists

Cardiovascular effect

Sublingual nifedipine was frequently given in the past for hypertensive emergencies; however, reports of increased ischemic events and mortality curtailed its use, primarily because of an unpredictable drop in blood pressure [29]. Nicardipine has gained popularity as a parenteral antihypertensive agent for managing postoperative hypertension and hypertensive crisis in the past decade, particularly in patients with brain injury. Nicardipine, a second-generation dihydropyridine calcium channel blocker, is structurally similar to nifedipine. With the addition of a tertiary amine, nicardipine is highly lipophilic and readily crosses the blood-brain barrier (BBB). Because of its chemical structure, the salt form of nicardipine is more water-soluble than nifedipine, which makes the intravenous preparation possible. Like other calcium channel blockers, nicardipine inhibits the influx of calcium into cardiac and smooth muscle cells, causing arteriolar vasodilation without a negative inotropic effect. The dose of nicardipine is independent of body weight, and the onset of action is within 5 to 10 minutes. Nicardipine has a relatively short duration of action (approximately 15 minutes) because of its rapid redistribution [57]. These pharmacokinetic characteristics allow for a titratable intravenous infusion.

Intravenous nicardipine has been shown to be as effective as nitroprusside in lowering blood pressure. A multicenter prospective study described a more rapid response to the goal blood pressure and less dosage adjustments with nicardipine compared with nitroprusside [58]. The incidence of hypotension was slightly higher with nitroprusside but not statistically significant. The efficacy of nicardipine compared with nitroprusside was also evaluated after surgery in patients who underwent carotid endarterectomy [59]. A more predictable therapeutic response (less variation in blood pressure) was observed with nicardipine than with nitroprusside. Fewer patients who received nicardipine compared with those who received nitroprusside required dosage adjustments. Results from these studies suggest that nicardipine is at least as effective as nitroprusside in lowering blood pressure and provides a more predictable response with less dosage adjustments.

Cerebrovascular effect

Nicardipine has generated great interest in its therapeutic role in treating cerebrovascular diseases, primarily because of its calcium blockade property and high cerebrovascular selectivity [60–62]. Because nicardipine is a vasodilator, one may question whether nicardipine increases CBF and adversely affects ICP like nitroprusside or nitroglycerin. Experimental and human data have indicated that nicardipine can increase CBF; however, it has little effect on ICP while lowering blood pressure. Unlike nitrovasodilators, nicardipine does not dilate all cerebral vessels, which may cause profound hypotension and cerebral ischemia. Gaab and coworkers [62] demonstrated that nicardipine dilates small-resistance arterioles with no significant changes in intracranial volume and ICP. Although MAP and CPP decreased significantly, CPP was within the critical level of autoregulation. Similarly, Nishiyama and colleagues [63] reported that nicardipine infusion in patients with ICH was safe and effective despite a slight decrease in CPP. The reported CPP was 99 $\pm$ 17 mm Hg at baseline, 75 $\pm$ 14 mm Hg at 24 hours of infusion, and 73 $\pm$ 15 mm Hg at 72 hours of infusion. No negative clinical consequences were observed with the nicardipine infusion in this study. As described previously, Powers and coworkers [25] also reported that nicardipine effectively reduced blood pressure up to 20% from baseline in patients with ICH without compromising autoregulation. In our own experience, nicardipine produced a moderate reduction in blood pressure and required less dosage adjustments and less additional antihypertensive agents compared with labetalol in patients with stroke [64].

In addition to the safety data in cerebral hemodynamics, nicardipine has been investigated for its potential neuroprotective effect. Because calcium plays an important role in propagating free oxygen radicals and subsequent neuronal injury after stroke, it is intuitive to speculate that a calcium antagonist may potentially attenuate further insult and improve neurologic recovery [65,66]. Earlier studies in spontaneous hypertensive rats suggested that nicardipine reduced neuronal cell death; however, current data supporting the neuroprotective effect of nicardipine are scarce. Future research is needed to determine the neuroprotective role of nicardipine.

Therapeutic implications

Nicardipine is an effective antihypertensive agent and has been used for hypertensive emergency. In addition to its effectiveness, studies have shown that nicardipine is easy to titrate and produces less variability while lowering blood pressure. Furthermore, it may have a pivotal role in treating hypertensive-related neurologic disorders because of its favorable cerebral hemodynamic effects.

Renin-angiotensin system blockade

Cardiovascular effect

The renin-angiotensin cascade has been known to contribute to the hypertensive state. Angiotensin-converting enzyme inhibitors (ACEIs) have been used in the treatment of chronic hypertension and congestive heart failure for many years. These agents are thought to be effective for hypertension via several mechanisms: (1) increasing concentrations of the local vasodilator bradykinin, (2) decreasing concentrations of angiotensin II, and (3) inhibiting the local vascular effects of angiotensin II. In patients with hypertension, ACEIs decrease total peripheral resistance but cause little change in heart rate, cardiac output, or pulmonary occlusion pressures [67]. In patients with congestive heart failure, however, cardiac output may increase in response to the afterload reduction [68].

Cerebrovascular effect

The effect of captopril on CBF has been extensively studied in rats and human beings. In general, studies that have evaluated renin-angiotensin system (RAS) blockade using ACEIs have shown increases in CBF with a shift in the autoregulatory curve [69–75]. This is in contrast to the direct vasodilators, which increase CBF and inhibit cerebral autoregulation.

In normotensive or spontaneously hypertensive rats, intravenously administered captopril shifts the upper (by 50–60 mm Hg) and lower (by 20–30 mm Hg) limits of the autoregulatory curve, and subsequently shortens the plateau of the curve by 20 to 40 mm Hg [72]. The mechanism by which ACEIs affect CBF is via inhibition of angiotensin II–mediated vascular tone in the large cerebral arteries while the small-resistance vessels constrict [76,77]. Therefore, in response to blood pressure decreases, these vessels dilate so that there is less capacity for vasoconstriction when the blood pressure is elevated. In patients with heart failure, captopril resulted in a reduction of blood pressure with no change in CBF [71] or an increase in CBF [69], suggesting an acute shift of the autoregulatory curve toward lower pressure. In patients with recent ischemic cerebral infarcts (2–7 days), the use of ACEIs reduced blood pressure without adversely affecting middle CBF velocity or global CBF in patients with and without carotid artery disease [70,74,75,78,79].

The effects of ACEIs on ICP have not been extensively studied. In patients with normal pressure hydrocephalus, captopril reduced MAP by 16 mm Hg without any effects on CBF or ICP [80]. There are currently no studies published evaluating patients with altered intracranial compliance and subsequent effects of

ACEIs on ICP, although with their effects on CBF, there may be a potential for increases in ICP in these patients.

The use of angiotensin receptor blocking agents (ARBs) has recently been investigated. The Acute Candesartan Cilexetil Therapy in Stroke Survivors Trial (ACCESS) compared the use of candesartan (4–16 mg) with acute (< 72 hours) versus delayed (> 7 days) initiation of therapy in 342 hypertensive (>180/105 mm Hg) patients with AIS [81]. The study was halted prematurely because of a significant reduction in the secondary end point (combined death, recurrent stroke, cardiac events, and dependency at 2 months; OR = 0.475, 95% CI, 0.252–0.895). The primary end point (death and disability at 3 months) was unchanged, however. There were no adverse cerebral effects reported with the acute use of this agent. Nazir and coworkers [82] observed that losartan could safely be introduced within 2 to 7 days of mild stroke in patients with hypertension and significant carotid disease without affecting global CBF or rCBF.

The use of agents affecting the RAS may extend beyond their blood pressure lowering properties. This system may adversely influence fibrinolytic balance, vascular endothelial function, and vascular inflammation, which are all key components of atherosclerotic progression and subsequent adverse vascular outcomes. Studies have suggested that ACEIs and ARBs may have favorable effects on various substances, including plasminogen activator inhibitor-1, endothelin-1, nitric oxide, vascular cell adhesion molecule-1, and C-reactive protein [83]. In clinical trials of antihypertensive therapy, however, monotherapy with ACEIs has failed to prevent primary stroke beyond their general effects on blood pressure [84,85]. In contrast, studies like the Losartan Intervention for Endpoint Reduction in Hypertension (LIFE) study have shown that the ARB losartan significantly prevented primary stroke compared with atenolol [86]. Some investigators have hypothesized that ARBs (which increase angiotensin II levels and stimulate the angiotensin type-2 receptor) have superior cerebroprotective properties compared with ACEIs [87]. In gerbils, at comparable blood pressure lowering effects, preadministration of an ARB had a lower incidence of mortality than preadministration of an ACEI. When the ACEI and the ARB were administered together, however, no reduction in the incidence of mortality was observed [88]. Therefore, ARBs may have superior mechanisms of action compared with ACEIs in that they inhibit the angiotensin type-1 receptor–mediated proatherothrombotic effects and enhance the angiotensin type-2 receptor–mediated cerebroprotection by increasing the generation of angiotensin II. Because ACEIs reduce circulating angiotensin II concentrations and subsequent angiotensin type-2 receptor cerebroprotection, their effects in blunting the proatherothrombotic effects mediated by the angiotensin type-1 receptor may be mitigated.

Activation of vascular angiotensin type-2 receptor has been shown to induce vasodilation by local synthesis of nitric oxide and prostacyclin. In the ischemic brain, there is overexpression of angiotensin type-2 receptors [89]; thus, collateral circulation may increase in ischemic areas. Chronic pretreatment and posttreatment with angiotensin type-1 receptor blocking agents in the rat brain improved neurologic outcome, infarct volume, and cerebral edema after cerebral ischemia

[90–95]. The results of the ACCESS study suggest that the use of ARBs is safe during the acute period, and a study is warranted to evaluate the potential vascular protective mechanisms associated with these agents acutely.

Therapeutic implications

There are many different agents that are available orally. Enalaprilat is currently the only available intravenous ACEI available in the United States, whereas an intravenous formulation of ARB is currently unavailable. The use of ACEIs or ARBs for the treatment of acute hypertension after stroke may seem appealing; however, the only intravenous agent available is associated with some disadvantages that may limit the widespread use of this agent acutely. Enalaprilat has an onset of action within 15 minutes; however, the duration of action is 12 to 24 hours. Furthermore, Hirshcl and coworkers [96] demonstrated that the degree of blood pressure reduction associated with this agent is related to the pretreatment concentration of angiotensin II and plasma renin activity. Because of the unpredictability of the response and long duration of action, the routine use of this agent to lower blood pressure acutely after an acute cerebrovascular event cannot be recommended. Future studies may show a neuroprotective effect of these agents; thus, ACEIs or ARBs may become part of the treatment regimen outside of their blood pressure lowering properties.

Other agents

Fenoldopam

Fenoldopam is a peripheral dopamine-1 receptor agonist, with its antihypertensive effects attributable to a combination of direct vasodilation and renal-arterial dilation with natriuresis [97]. It does not bind to the dopamine-2 receptors or β-adrenergic receptors or possess α-adrenergic agonist effects; however, it is an α_2-antagonist [30]. Therapeutic doses of fenoldopam reduce SBP and DBP, with an increase in heart rate proportional to this decrease. Renal vascular resistance decreases, whereas renal blood flow and glomerular filtration rate increase. These effects seem to be greater in the hypertensive population. Fenoldopam is poorly soluble in lipids, does not cross the BBB, and has no CNS effects in patients with an intact BBB [98].

Dopamine has a wide spectrum of effects that could ultimately affect CBF. The effects of fenoldopam on cerebral circulation are poorly defined in patients with acute stroke. In nine normotensive healthy volunteers (with autoregulation presumed to be intact), fenoldopam-induced hypotension significantly decreased global CBF [99]. Hennes and Jantzen [100] evaluated the effects of fenoldopam on ICP under conditions of normal and increased intracranial elastance in pigs. Fenoldopam did not increase ICP when ICP was normal; however, under conditions of elevated ICP, fenoldopam resulted in increases in ICP, suggesting a shift in the volume-pressure curve to the right. This study did not find that fenoldopam affected cerebral autoregulation or carbon dioxide reactivity [100].

Reports on this experimental model would suggest that fenoldopam should be used in caution in patients with altered intracranial compliance.

The onset of clinical effects is rapid (within 5 minutes), and effects disappear within 30 minutes from termination of the infusion. Common adverse effects include headache, flushing, tachycardia, dizziness, and a dose-related increase in intraocular pressure. The clinical utility of this agent in patients with cerebrovascular disease is limited until further information is available to assess its effects acutely in these patients.

Hydralazine

Hydralazine is a direct-acting smooth muscle relaxant that causes vasodilation to a greater extent in arteries than in veins. It acts by interference with vascular smooth muscle calcium transport and has also been shown to generate nitric oxide [101]. In animals without intracranial pathologic changes, small increases in ICP with no alteration or small increases in CBF have been reported [102]. In patients with severe brain injury, administration of hydralazine resulted in increases in ICP with defective or absent cerebral autoregulation [103,104]. CBF remained stable or slightly increased in these patients despite the increases in ICP. Hydralazine causes reflex stimulation of the sympathetic nervous system, with increases in ICP in patients with head injury [105]. This effect can be blunted by coadministration of β-receptor antagonists. The onset of action of hydralazine is within 15 minutes, with a half-life of 3 hours; however, the half-time of its effect on blood pressure is approximately 100 hours [106]. Because of its prolonged and unpredictable antihypertensive effects in addition to the effects reported on the cerebrovasculature, hydralazine should be avoided in patients with acute stroke.

Summary

Controversy surrounds the ideal management of blood pressure during the acute phase of stroke. The primary goal in acute blood pressure management in these patients is to avoid further insults to the brain and minimize neurologic deficit. Evidence suggests that the initial elevation of blood pressure may be a protective mechanism to ensure adequate blood perfusion to the brain. Particularly in ischemic stroke, elevated blood pressure may be essential to the penumbra area, where blood flow is pressure dependent. More aggressive blood pressure lowering can be applied in ICH compared with AIS, because evidence suggests the absence of a periclot penumbra; however, precipitous drops in blood pressure may still induce ischemia and should be avoided. Conversely, studies also demonstrate that severe hypertension may exacerbate brain edema or induce a hemorrhagic event. Although debate continues, many practitioners think that it is necessary to treat severe hypertension with a moderate lowering of blood pressure [12,13,107].

When treatment is deemed necessary, blood pressure should be lowered cautiously during the first 24 hours so as to avoid further ischemia to the brain tissue. Therefore, a short-acting, titratable, and predictable agent should be used. Nitroprusside has been widely used in managing hypertensive crisis and is recommended in current guidelines [12,13,107]; however, its potential effect on increasing ICP cannot be ignored. In addition, cyanide or thiocyanate toxicity is a major concern and difficult to diagnose, especially in patients with impaired mental status after stroke. Based on limited clinical evidence, labetalol and nicardipine seem to produce moderate and predictable reductions in blood pressure with minimal effect on the cerebrovasculature. Currently, there are no comparative trials of these two agents to demonstrate equivalency or superiority in the acute setting. Future comparative studies should evaluate clinical end points, such as time to goal blood pressure, degree of blood pressure reduction, and safety. There are many unanswered questions related to blood pressure management after AIS or ICH. Large clinical trials are necessary to delineate the threshold for initiation of therapy, the appropriate degree of blood pressure reduction and the resultant impact on clinical outcomes, and the timing of acute blood pressure management in these patients.

References

[1] American Heart Association. Heart disease and stroke statistics—2005 update. Dallas (TX): American Heart Association; 2005.

[2] Leonardi-Bee J, Bath PM, Phillips SJ, et al. Blood pressure and clinical outcomes in the International Stroke Trial. Stroke 2002;33(5):1315–20.

[3] Britton M, Carlsson A, de Faire U. Blood pressure course in patients with acute stroke and matched controls. Stroke 1986;17(5):861–4.

[4] Wallace JD, Levy LL. Blood pressure after stroke. JAMA 1981;246(19):2177–80.

[5] Lang EW, Lagopoulos J, Griffith J, et al. Cerebral vasomotor reactivity testing in head injury: the link between pressure and flow. J Neurol Neurosurg Psychiatry 2003;74(8):1053–9.

[6] Astrup J, Siesjo BK, Symon L. Thresholds in cerebral ischemia-the ischemic penumbra. Stroke 1981;12(6):726–30.

[7] Eames PJ, Blake MJ, Dawson SL, et al. Dynamic cerebral autoregulation and beat to beat blood pressure control are impaired in acute ischaemic stroke. J Neurol Neurosurg Psychiatry 2002; 72(4):467–72.

[8] Okumura K, Ohya Y, Maehara A, et al. Effects of blood pressure levels on case fatality after acute stroke. J Hypertens 2005;23(6):1217–23.

[9] Rordorf G, Koroshetz WJ, Ezzeddine MA, et al. A pilot study of drug-induced hypertension for treatment of acute stroke. Neurology 2001;56(9):1210–3.

[10] Chalela JA, Dunn B, Todd JW, et al. Induced hypertension improves cerebral blood flow in acute ischemic stroke. Neurology 2005;64(11):1979.

[11] Willmot M, Leonardi-Bee J, Bath PM. High blood pressure in acute stroke and subsequent outcome: a systematic review. Hypertension 2004;43(1):18–24.

[12] Adams Jr HP, Adams RJ, Brott T, et al. Guidelines for the early management of patients with ischemic stroke: a scientific statement from the Stroke Council of the American Stroke Association. Stroke 2003;34(4):1056–83.

[13] Adams H, Adams R, Del Zoppo G, et al. Guidelines for the early management of patients with ischemic stroke: 2005 guidelines update: a scientific statement from the Stroke Council of the American Heart Association/American Stroke Association. Stroke 2005;36(4):916–23.

[14] Eastern Stroke and Coronary Heart Disease Collaborative Research Group. Blood pressure, cholesterol, and stroke in Eastern Asia. Lancet 1998;352(9143):1801–7.

[15] Dandapani BK, Suzuki S, Kelley RE, et al. Relation between blood pressure and outcome in intracerebral hemorrhage. Stroke 1995;26(1):21–4.

[16] Kazui S, Minematsu K, Yamamoto H, et al. Predisposing factors to enlargement of spontaneous intracerebral hematoma. Stroke 1997;28(12):2370–5.

[17] Leira R, Davalos A, Silva Y, et al. Early neurologic deterioration in intracerebral hemorrhage: predictors and associated factors. Neurology 2004;63(3):461–7.

[18] Ohwaki K, Yano E, Nagashima H, et al. Blood pressure management in acute intracerebral hemorrhage: relationship between elevated blood pressure and hematoma enlargement. Stroke 2004;35(6):1364–7.

[19] Fujii Y, Takeuchi S, Sasaki O, et al. Multivariate analysis of predictors of hematoma enlargement in spontaneous intracerebral hemorrhage. Stroke 1998;29(6):1160–6.

[20] Qureshi AI, Wilson DA, Hanley DF, et al. Pharmacologic reduction of mean arterial pressure does not adversely affect regional cerebral blood flow and intracranial pressure in experimental intracerebral hemorrhage. Crit Care Med 1999;27(5):965–71.

[21] Kuwata N, Kuroda K, Funayama M, et al. Dysautoregulation in patients with hypertensive intracerebral hemorrhage. A SPECT study. Neurosurg Rev 1995;18(4):237–45.

[22] Carhuapoma JR, Wang PY, Beauchamp NJ, et al. Diffusion-weighted MRI and proton MR spectroscopic imaging in the study of secondary neuronal injury after intracerebral hemorrhage. Stroke 2000;31(3):726–32.

[23] Kidwell CS, Saver JL, Mattiello J, et al. Diffusion-perfusion MR evaluation of perihematomal injury in hyperacute intracerebral hemorrhage. Neurology 2001;57(9):1611–7.

[24] Zazulia AR, Diringer MN, Videen TO, et al. Hypoperfusion without ischemia surrounding acute intracerebral hemorrhage. J Cereb Blood Flow Metab 2001;21(7):804–10.

[25] Powers WJ, Zazulia AR, Videen TO, et al. Autoregulation of cerebral blood flow surrounding acute (6 to 22 hours) intracerebral hemorrhage. Neurology 2001;57(1):18–24.

[26] Schellinger PD, Fiebach JB, Hoffmann K, et al. Stroke MRI in intracerebral hemorrhage: is there a perihemorrhagic penumbra? Stroke 2003;34(7):1674–9.

[27] Intensive blood pressure reduction in acute cerebral haemorrhage. NCT00226096. Available at: www.clinicaltrial.gov. Accessed January 2006.

[28] Chobanian AV, Bakris GL, Black HR, et al. Seventh report of the Joint National Committee on Prevention, Detection, Evaluation, and Treatment of High Blood Pressure. Hypertension 2003; 42(6):1206–52.

[29] Erstad BL, Barletta JF. Treatment of hypertension in the perioperative patient. Ann Pharmacother 2000;34(1):66–79.

[30] Varon J, Marik PE. The diagnosis and management of hypertensive crises. Chest 2000; 118(1):214–27.

[31] Abdelwahab W, Frishman W, Landau A. Management of hypertensive urgencies and emergencies. J Clin Pharmacol 1995;35(8):747–62.

[32] Sipe EK, Trienski TL, Porter JM. Cyanide toxicity in the surgical intensive care unit: a case report. Am Surg 2001;67(7):684–6.

[33] Alaniz C, Watts B. Monitoring cyanide toxicity in patients receiving nitroprusside therapy. Ann Pharmacother 2005;39(2):388–9.

[34] Cottrell JE, Casthely P, Brodie JD, et al. Mechanism and prevention of tachyphylaxis and cyanide toxicosis after nitroprusside-induced hypotension. Surg Forum 1978;29:308–10.

[35] Cottrell JE, Patel K, Turndorf H, et al. Intracranial pressure changes induced by sodium nitroprusside in patients with intracranial mass lesions. J Neurosurg 1978;48(3):329–31.

[36] Griswold WR, Reznik V, Mendoza SA. Nitroprusside-induced intracranial hypertension. JAMA 1981;246(23):2679–80.

[37] Anile C, Zanghi F, Bracali A, et al. Sodium nitroprusside and intracranial pressure. Acta Neurochir (Wien) 1981;58(3–4):203–11.

[38] Larsen R, Teichmann J, Hilfiker O, et al. Nitroprusside-hypotension: cerebral blood flow and cerebral oxygen consumption in neurosurgical patients. Acta Anaesthesiol Scand 1982; 26(4):327–30.

[39] Griffiths DP, Cummins BH, Greenbaum R, et al. Cerebral blood flow and metabolism during hypotension induced with sodium nitroprusside. Br J Anaesth 1974;46(9):671–9.

[40] Fitch W, Ferguson GG, Sengupta D, et al. Autoregulation of cerebral blood flow during controlled hypotension in baboons. J Neurol Neurosurg Psychiatry 1976;39(10):1014–22.
[41] Stoyka WW, Schutz H. The cerebral response to sodium nitroprusside and trimethaphan controlled hypotension. Can Anaesth Soc J 1975;22(3):275–83.
[42] Turner JM, Powell D, Gibson RM, et al. Intracranial pressure changes in neurosurgical patients during hypotension induced with sodium nitroprusside or trimetaphan. Br J Anaesth 1977;49(5):419–25.
[43] Ivankovich AD, Miletich DJ, Albrecht RF, et al. Sodium nitroprusside and cerebral blood flow in the anesthetized and unanesthetized goat. Anesthesiology 1976;44(1):21–6.
[44] Crockard HA, Brown FD, Mullan JF. Effects of trimethaphan and sodium nitroprusside on cerebral blood flow in rhesus monkeys. Acta Neurochir (Wien) 1976;35(1–3):85–9.
[45] Brown FD, Hanlon K, Crockard HA, et al. Effect of sodium nitroprusside on cerebral blood flow in conscious human beings. Surg Neurol 1977;7(2):67–70.
[46] Miller CL, Lampard DG, Griffiths RI, et al. Local cerebral blood flow and the electrocorticogram during sodium nitroprusside hypotension. Anaesth Intensive Care 1978;6(4):290–6.
[47] Miletich DJ, Gil KS, Albrecht RF, et al. Intracerebral blood flow distribution during hypotensive anesthesia in the goat. Anesthesiology 1980;53(3):210–4.
[48] Brown MJ. Vasodilator drugs: systemic and regional considerations. Anaesth Intensive Care 1980;8(3):310–7.
[49] Kistler JP, Lees RS, Candia G, et al. Intravenous nitroglycerin in experimental cerebral vasospasm. A preliminary report. Stroke 1979;10(1):26–9.
[50] Lagerkranser M. Effects of nitroglycerin on intracranial pressure and cerebral blood flow. Acta Anaesthesiol Scand Suppl 1992;97:34–6.
[51] Gagnon RL, Marsh ML, Smith RW, et al. Intracranial hypertension caused by nitroglycerin. Anesthesiology 1979;51(1):86–7.
[52] Ohar JM, Fowler AA, Selhorst JB, et al. Intravenous nitroglycerin-induced intracranial hypertension. Crit Care Med 1985;13(10):867–8.
[53] Griffith DN, James IM, Newbury PA, et al. The effect of beta-adrenergic receptor blocking drugs on cerebral blood flow. Br J Clin Pharmacol 1979;7(5):491–4.
[54] Olsen KS, Svendsen LB, Larsen FS, et al. Effect of labetalol on cerebral blood flow, oxygen metabolism and autoregulation in healthy humans. Br J Anaesth 1995;75(1):51–4.
[55] Patel RV, Kertland HR, Jahns BE, et al. Labetalol: response and safety in critically ill hemorrhagic stroke patients. Ann Pharmacother 1993;27(2):180–1.
[56] Larive L, Rhoney D, Parker D, et al. Acute blood pressure management in ischemic and hemorrhagic stroke [abstract 22]. Crit Care Med 2003;31(Suppl):S495.
[57] Haas CE, LeBlanc JM. Acute postoperative hypertension: a review of therapeutic options. Am J Health Syst Pharm 2004;61(16):1661–73 [quiz: 74–5].
[58] Halpern NA, Goldberg M, Neely C, et al. Postoperative hypertension: a multicenter, prospective, randomized comparison between intravenous nicardipine and sodium nitroprusside. Crit Care Med 1992;20(12):1637–43.
[59] Dorman T, Thompson DA, Breslow MJ, et al. Nicardipine versus nitroprusside for breakthrough hypertension following carotid endarterectomy. J Clin Anesth 2001;13(1):16–9.
[60] Sabbatini M, Bellagamba G, Casado A, et al. Protective effect of treatment with nicardipine on cerebrovascular tree of spontaneously hypertensive rats. Clin Exp Hypertens 2001;23(1–2):143–55.
[61] Suzuki S, Ohtsuka S, Ishikawa K, et al. Effects of nicardipine on coronary, vertebral and renal arterial flows in patients with essential hypertension. Hypertens Res 2003;26(3):193–9.
[62] Gaab MR, Czech T, Korn A. Intracranial effects of nicardipine. Br J Clin Pharmacol 1985;20(Suppl 1):67S–74S.
[63] Nishiyama T, Yokoyama T, Matsukawa T, et al. Continuous nicardipine infusion to control blood pressure after evacuation of acute cerebral hemorrhage. Can J Anaesth 2000;47(12):1196–201.
[64] DeRyke-Liu X, Parker D, Rhoney D. Nicardipine vs. labetalol for acute blood pressure control after stroke. Crit Care Med 2005;33:A103.

ELSEVIER
SAUNDERS

Crit Care Clin 22 (2006) 245–253

CRITICAL
CARE
CLINICS

Corticosteroid Replacement in Critically Ill Patients

Judith Jacobi, PharmD

Pharmacy Department Methodist Hospital/Clarian Health Partners, AG401, 1701 North Senate Boulevard, Indianapolis, IN 46202, USA

Corticosteroids are a standard treatment in many disease states with an inflammatory cause. The hormonal contribution of corticosteroids has gained a prominent role in the care of many critically ill patients, including patients with septic shock. Controversy exists regarding the optimal method to identify patients likely to benefit from corticosteroid therapy and the optimal treatment regimen. These issues are reviewed and discussed in this article.

Steroid physiology

Corticosteroids are produced by the adrenal glands, which are located superior to the kidneys in the extraperitoneal area. The adrenal glands produce several hormones. The adrenal medulla secretes catecholamines. This portion occupies approximately 10% of the adrenal gland. The zona glomerulosa occupies 15% of the adrenal cortex and produces mineralocorticoids—precursors of aldosterone. The zona fasciculata is the largest portion, composing 60% of the cortex. This region produces basal and stimulated glucocorticoids, mainly cortisol. The zona reticularis, 25% of the adrenal cortex, produces testosterone and estradiol.

Cortisol is produced after stepwise release of corticotropin-releasing hormone by the hypothalamus and subsequent release of adrenocorticotropic hormone (ACTH) from the anterior pituitary. The ACTH stimulates release of cortisol from the adrenal cortex and aldosterone and androgens. Cortisol activity regulates its own production by providing negative feedback to the hypothalamus and pituitary. Norepinephrine seems to stimulate the release of ACTH directly. In-

E-mail address: jjacobi@clarian.org

doi:10.1016/j.ccc.2006.02.007 *criticalcare.theclinics.com*

flammatory mediators, such as interleukin-1, interleukin-6, and tumor necrosis factor, stimulate the release of corticotropin-releasing hormone, leading to cortisol secretion in response to stress.

Basal cortisol production is estimated to be 8 to 25 mg in a 24-hour period, although production can be increased sixfold in severe illness or injury. Cortisol production is typically diurnal, but this characteristic is lost during stress-related overproduction. Cortisol has a half-life of 70 to 120 minutes and is eliminated primarily by hepatic metabolism and glomerular filtration. Glucocorticoid clearance is enhanced by compounds that stimulate hepatic metabolism, including phenytoin, rifampin, and phenobarbital, and changes in metabolic rate, as in hyperthyroidism. Glucocorticoid production is impaired by mitotane, aminoglutethimide, etomidate, ketoconazole, megestrol, and possibly high-dose fluconazole [1]. Glucocorticoid clearance is reduced by estrogens, liver disease, age, pregnancy, hypothyroidism, anorexia nervosa, and malnutrition.

Glucocorticoids are bound primarily to circulating corticosteroid-binding globulin (CBG), but also to albumin and α1-acid glycoprotein, with approximately 10% in the free, biologically active form. The clinical significance of changes in CBG and subsequent changes in free cortisol concentrations has been poorly defined because of technical limitations in the ability to assay free cortisol clinically. Concentrations of CBG decrease rapidly in critically ill patients, increasing free cortisol concentrations and the calculated free cortisol index [2]. The free cortisol index (cortisol concentration [μmol/L] ÷ CBG [mg/mL] × 100) may reflect free cortisol concentrations more accurately, but its clinical utility is unproven in critically ill patients [3]. Free cortisol concentrations and the free cortisol index are elevated in response to acute stress despite low total cortisol concentrations and reduced concentrations of serum proteins, such as albumin and CBG [2,4]. Clinical trials of adrenal function primarily have reported total cortisol concentrations and may overestimate the rate of adrenal insufficiency in critically ill patients with abnormal binding proteins.

Free cortisol is active at the receptor level. Cortisol is liberated from CBG at sites of inflammation by neutrophil elastase. Local cortisol concentrations also are increased by inflammatory cytokines through changes in peripheral metabolism and receptor affinity [5].

Adrenal insufficiency

Adrenal insufficiency can be primary or secondary in origin. Primary adrenal insufficiency (Addison's disease) results from greater than 90% destruction of the adrenal cortex with deficiencies in cortisol, aldosterone, and androgens. Adrenal damage with a rapid onset of symptoms can follow thrombosis, hemorrhage from coagulopathy or severe sepsis or necrosis after ischemia. Septic shock with disseminated intravascular coagulopathy is the most common cause of adrenal hemorrhage. A slower onset of adrenal insufficiency may be the result of damage from conditions such as HIV, amyloidosis, autoimmune adrenalitis, congenital hypoplasia, metastatic neoplasia, or adrenal infections. Stressful situations that increase the demand for cortisol may trigger adrenal insufficiency when the ability to increase cortisol production is limited.

Symptoms of adrenal insufficiency may be difficult to differentiate from other critical illnesses and include truncal pain, fever, shaking chills, hypotension and shock, and abdominal rigidity or rebound. Dehydration, hyponatremia, hyperkalemia, and elevated blood urea nitrogen are common. Hypoglycemia, anorexia, headache, vertigo, vomiting, rash, and psychiatric symptoms also may occur. Failure to recognize and treat severe adrenal insufficiency (addisonian crisis) may be fatal, with death in 6 to 48 hours.

Diagnostic clues to the presence of adrenal insufficiency in critically ill patients include persistent hypotension despite adequate volume resuscitation, especially with a hyperdynamic circulation and low systemic vascular resistance. Patients with severe sepsis and septic shock as a source of ongoing inflammation commonly have been evaluated for adrenal insufficiency. Secondary adrenal insufficiency is the result of pituitary or hypothalamic abnormalities, including empty sella syndrome, tumors, hypopituitarism (medical or surgical), sarcoidosis, head trauma with pituitary trauma, and postpartum pituitary necrosis, or most often exogenous glucocorticoid use. Glucocorticoid-induced suppression of the hypothalamic-pituitary-adrenal axis may be the result of therapy via the oral, intravenous, inhaled, intranasal, or topical routes. Short courses (5 days) of prednisone suppress the hypothalamic-pituitary-adrenal axis for 5 days after discontinuation [6]. Long-term glucocorticoid use produces adrenal cortical atrophy as a result of chronic suppression of ACTH production, requiring variable recovery times of up to 1 year [7]. Drugs that reduce cortisol production or increase metabolism also may cause secondary insufficiency, as previously discussed.

Clinical presentation of secondary adrenal insufficiency can be difficult to distinguish from primary insufficiency, although aldosterone secretion is preserved, so sodium and potassium abnormalities are uncommon. A third syndrome has been reported in critically ill patients, termed *relative* or *functional adrenal insufficiency* [8]. A hypoadrenal state is present without clearly defined defects in the hypothalamic-pituitary-adrenal axis. This syndrome has been difficult to define based on serum cortisol concentrations because the cortisol production may be inadequate to control the inflammatory response or meet an elevated metabolic demand.

Laboratory diagnosis of adrenal insufficiency

The standard for assessment of cortisol production is the high-dose corticotropin-stimulation test. After obtaining blood for a baseline cortisol concentration, the patient is given a 250-μg injection of synthetic ACTH (cosyntropin). Cortisol concentrations are measured 30 and 60 minutes later. An increase in cortisol to a value of 18 μg/dL or greater ($\geq$500 nmol/L) rules out adrenal insufficiency in a nonstressed patient [9]. (To convert values, multiply μg/dL $\times$ 27.7 to equal nmol/L.)

The corticotropin-stimulation test may be done at any time of the day. A subnormal change in cortisol suggests the presence of primary or secondary adrenal insufficiency, although values of 15 μg/dL have been reported in healthy persons. This test shows a high degree of sensitivity and specificity in patients with primary adrenal insufficiency using a threshold value of 15 μg/dL, although most patients achieve a cortisol value less than 10 μg/dL [9]. Patients with equivocal results may improve clinically after glucocorticoid therapy.

Secondary adrenal insufficiency is similarly diagnosed with the high-dose corticotropin–stimulation test. Failure to achieve a cortisol concentration of at least 18 μg/dL increases the likelihood that the patient has secondary adrenal insufficiency, especially when clinical suspicion is high. This test is less sensitive to rule out secondary adrenal insufficiency, and low-dose corticotropin testing has been proposed using 1-μg doses of cosyntropin to produce a more physiologic ACTH level; however, clinical trials have failed to show a significant difference between the two methods [9]. The low-dose corticotropin–stimulation test is complicated by the need to perform accurate dilutions to achieve a reliable product for intravenous administration, with carefully timed venous sampling.

Adrenal insufficiency in critical illness

Although primary and secondary adrenal insufficiency may be found in critically ill patients, the diagnosis with corticotropin-stimulation testing is more challenging. Cortisol concentrations should be elevated in response to critical illness, although the degree varies with the disease and severity of illness. Extremely high (>34 μg/dL) and extremely low (<25 μg/dL) total cortisol concentrations have been associated with a poor prognosis in septic shock patients [10,11]. As discussed previously, reduced CBG complicates interpretation of total cortisol concentrations. In addition, changes in tissue resistance to cortisol and local release of free cortisol may determine whether clinical symptoms of insufficiency are present. Interpretation of current literature is complicated further by the use of etomidate for intubation of many critically ill patients, an agent that lowers cortisol concentrations and synthesis for at least 24 hours, leading to recommendations against the use of this agent in patients with sepsis [12–14].

The laboratory diagnosis and treatment of adrenal insufficiency in critical illness are complex and challenging. A cortisol concentration less than 15 μg/dL has been suggested to identify patients with clinical features of corticosteroid insufficiency or who would benefit from replacement therapy [5]. Other investigators have suggested, however, that a septic shock patient receiving vasopressor therapy should have a baseline cortisol concentration greater than 25 μg/dL when measured within 48 hours of admission [15].

To solve the problem of variable basal concentrations, corticotropin-stimulation testing has been advocated as the standard for diagnosis of adrenal insufficiency in critically ill patients. Failure to increase the cortisol concentration at least 9 μg/dL to a value greater than 20 μg/dL has been associated with lack of response to catecholamines or increased mortality in critically ill patients [10,16,17]. Timing of the test also may be important with a different response shown within 24 hours and 48 hours of assessment [18]. There is disagreement on the threshold basal concentration or change in cortisol necessary to make the diagnosis, leading to a call for a consensus definition of relative adrenal insufficiency in critically ill patients.

Glucocorticoid replacement

Pharmaceutical glucocorticoids, prednisone and cortisone, are prodrugs that require metabolism for conversion to active compounds, prednisolone and cortisol. Hydrocortisone and methylprednisolone are preferentially used. The potency and elimination rate of the glucocorticoids vary (Table 1) [19]. Periprocedural stress dosing depends on the duration and invasiveness of the procedure. A single extra dose before minor procedures or with a limited medical illness may be adequate, whereas major surgery with general anesthesia should be preceded by 100 to 150 mg of hydrocortisone on the day of the procedure with rapid tapering over 1 to 2 days to the patients usual dose (Table 2).

A variety of doses have been used as replacement therapy in critically ill patients depending on the degree of surgical stress (see Table 2). A low dosage used for steroid replacement is 200 to 300 mg of hydrocortisone equivalent per day, administered as intermittent doses or via continuous infusion [20–23]. One study also included 50 μg of fludrocortisone daily replacement by mouth [17]. Prednisolone, 7.5 mg/d intravenously (5 mg in the morning and 2.5 mg at night), also has been studied [24]. Early trials showed that high-dose steroid therapy methylprednisolone 30 mg/kg is detrimental and should not be a component of severe sepsis therapy [22,25].

The duration of hydrocortisone replacement therapy has varied in clinical trials from 5 to 7 days to 10 days or may depend on the clinical response to therapy. Tapering regimens have been used in some clinical trials [20]. If symptoms of

Table 1
Systemic glucocorticoid comparison

Glucocorticoid	Equivalent dose (mg)	Half-life (min)
Cortisone	25	30
Hydrocortisone	20	90
Prednisone	5	60
Prednisolone	5	200
Triamcinolone	4	300
Methylprednisolone	4	180
Dexamethasone	0.75	100–300

Adapted from Gums JG, Tovar JM. Adrenal gland disorders. In: DiPiro JT, Talbert RT, Yee GC, editors. Pharmacotherapy: a pathophysiologic approach. 6th edition. New York: McGraw-Hill Companies; 2005. p. 1403.

Table 2
Guidelines for adrenal supplementation therapy*

Medical or surgical stress	Corticosteroid dosage
Minor	
Inguinal hernia repair Colonoscopy Mild febrile illness Mild-moderate nausea vomiting Gastroenteritis	25 mg hydrocortisone *or* 5 mg methylprednisolone intravenously on day of procedure only
Moderate	
Open cholecystectomy Hemicolectomy Significant febrile illness Pneumonia Severe gastroenteritis	50–75 mg hydrocortisone *or* 10–15 mg methylprednisolone intravenously on day of procedure; taper over 1–2 days to usual dose
Severe	
Major cardiothoracic surgery Whipple procedure Liver resection Pancreatitis	100–150 mg hydrocortisone *or* 20–30 mg methylprednisolone intravenously on day of procedure; taper over 1–2 days to usual dose
Critically ill	
Sepsis-induced hypotension or shock	50–100 mg hydrocortisone intravenously *or* 50 mg intravenously every 6 to 8 hours 0.18 mg/kg/h infusion plus 50 μg fludrocortisone orally per day until shock resolves; duration 5–10 days, then discontinue or taper (resume for recurrent shock)

* Data are based on extrapolation from the literature, expert opinion, and clinical experience. Patients receiving prednisone doses ≤5 mg/d should receive their usual dose without supplementation. Patients receiving prednisone >5 mg/d should receive the above therapy in addition to their usual maintenance dose.

Adapted from Coursin DB, Wood KE. Corticosteroid supplementation for adrenal insufficiency. JAMA 2002;287(2):236–40.

hypotension or shock recur after steroid discontinuation, the regimen should be resumed at the prior dose and tapered, if no other cause is found.

Outcome of steroid replacement

Mortality reduction is the primary outcome measure for the use of steroids in septic shock, although a decrease in all-cause mortality at day 28 was not found with steroid replacement in a meta-analysis [20]. Inclusion of high-dose glucocorticoid trials may have influenced this result because more recent trials have shown a significant reduction in ICU mortality ($n = 425$; relative risk 0.83; 95% confidence interval [CI], 0.7–0.97). Evaluation of trials published after 1997 indicate a consistent and overall improvement in survival associated with glucocorticoid use (relative survival benefit 1.23; 95% CI, 1.01–1.5) [22]. These more recent trials used a consistent definition of sepsis and lower steroid doses than the trials before 1989. The most consistent finding with steroid replacement has been more rapid resolution of shock by day 7 compared with standard therapy (six trials, $n = 728$; relative risk 1.22; 95% CI, 1.06–1.4) and by day 28 in four additional trials [20]. A large confirmatory clinical trial of hydrocortisone replacement in septic shock is under way in Europe to assess the impact on 28-day mortality in patients who are nonresponders to ACTH (cortisol $\leq$9 μg/dL increase or failure to achieve >9 μg/dL) [26].

The mechanism by which steroids reduce or eliminate vasopressor requirements is likely multifaceted. A detailed report of the potential mechanisms is reviewed elsewhere [27]. Briefly, glucocorticoids bind to a glucocorticoid receptor that is complexed with heat-shock proteins in the cytoplasm. Glucocorticoid interaction with the glucocorticoid receptor releases heat-shock proteins, and the steroid forms a dimer with the glucocorticoid receptor. This complex reduces production of nuclear factor (NF)-κB and increases production of the inhibitor of NF-κB, leading to a reduced production of inflammatory cytokines. Most cytokine production is inhibited by glucocorticoids, including interleukin-2, interleukin-3, interleukin-5, γ-interferon, tumor necrosis factor, and a variety of chemokines. Eicosanoid inhibition reduces cyclooxygenase-2 and leukotriene C_4 activity. In addition, steroids prevent the release of platelet-activating factor and reduce nitric oxide production through inhibition of inducible nitric oxide synthetase. These and other effects can decrease inflammation, vasodilation, and the need for vasopressors. Low-dose steroids also produce chemical changes, such as a reduction in C-reactive protein, interleukin-6 plasma concentrations, and ex vivo lipopolysaccharide-stimulated production of interleukin-1 and interleukin-6 [21].

The adverse effect profile of short-term steroid therapy is limited; a meta-analysis found adverse events to be no different from control patients [20]. Clinical trials frequently report gastrointestinal bleeding, superinfections, and hyperglycemia. Other potential adverse effects include sodium and water retention, hypokalemia, and reduced wound healing, although these are not typically reported. The use of corticosteroids is a risk factor for ICU-acquired paresis, however [28].

Clinical benefits of low-dose steroids may occur in other critically ill patient populations without septic shock. Hydrocortisone infusion improved oxygenation, improved chest radiograph score, significantly reduced C-reactive protein, reduced multiple organ dysfunction syndrome score, and delayed septic shock in patients with severe community-acquired pneumonia [29]. Hydrocortisone also was associated with a reduction in length of hospital stay, but the authors suggest that a larger trial be performed before routine clinical use in community-acquired pneumonia. Data on the benefit of corticosteroid replacement in pediatric patients or patients with HIV are lacking, although the potential for adrenal insufficiency has been well described [30,31]. Trauma with hemorrhagic shock and ruptured abdominal aortic aneurysm surgery also has been found to impair adrenal reserve, although the clinical utility of corticosteroid therapy remains to be shown [16,32]. Although high-dose corticosteroids are not beneficial for early treatment of neurotrauma patients, adrenal insufficiency has been shown within 2 to 4 days of head injury, and a trial of low-dose hydrocortisone replacement therapy is under way [33,34].

Recommendations

Patients with septic shock should have a baseline cortisol concentration and ideally undergo corticotropin-stimulation testing with 1 μg or 250 μg. Although the definition of adrenal insufficiency remains to be fully elucidated, patients with an inadequate cortisol response (baseline <15-25 μg/dL and failure to increase cortisol by at least 9 μg/dL) benefit from glucocorticoid replacement. Hydrocortisone in total daily doses of 200 to 300 mg/d is recommended, with intermittent or continuous intravenous administration. The role of oral fludrocortisone replacement also remains inadequately defined, but fludrocortisone may be a desirable adjunct. Steroid therapy should continue for no more than 5 to 7 days, then be tapered as the patient improves, to achieve a total duration of 10 days.

References

[1] Albert SG, DeLeon J, Silverberg AB. Possible association between high-dose fluconazole and adrenal insufficiency in critically ill patients. Crit Care Med 2001;29:668–70.

[2] Beishuizen A, Thijs LG, Vermes I. Patterns of corticosteroid-binding globulin and the free cortisol index during septic shock and multitrauma. Intensive Care Med 2001;27:1584–91.

[3] Bonte HA, van den Hoven RJ, van der Sluijs Veer G, Vermes I. The use of free cortisol index for laboratory assessment of pituitary-adrenal function. Clin Chem Lab Med 1999;37:127–32.

[4] Hamrahian AH, Tawakalitu SO, Awafah BM. Measurements of serum free cortisol in critically ill patients. N Engl J Med 2004;350:1629–38.

[5] Cooper MS, Stewart PM. Corticosteroid insufficiency in acutely ill patients. N Engl J Med 2003;348:727–34.

[6] Streck WF, Lockwood DW. Pituitary adrenal recovery following short-term suppression with corticosteroids. Am J Med 1979;66:910–4.

[7] Lamberts SWJ, Bruining HA, DeJong FH. Corticosteroid therapy in severe illness. N Engl J Med 1997;337:1285–92.

[8] Ballaert PE. Stress doses of glucocorticoids in cathecholamine dependency: a new therapy for a new syndrome. Intensive Care Med 2000;26(1):3–5.

[9] Dorin RI, Qualls CR, Crapo LM. Diagnosis of adrenal insufficiency. Ann Intern Med 2003;139:194–204.

[10] Annane D, Sébille V, Troché G, et al. A 3-level prognostic classification in septic shock based on cortisol levels and cortisol response to corticotropin. JAMA 2000;283:1038–45.

[11] Marik PE, Zaloga GP. Adrenal insufficiency in the critically ill: a new look at an old problem. Chest 2002;122:1784–96.

[12] Absalom A, Pledger D, Kong A. Adrenocortical function in critically ill patients 24h after a single dose of etomidate. Anaesthesia 1999;54:861–7.

[13] Malerba G, Romano-Girard F, Cravoisy A, et al. Risk factors of relative adrenocortical deficiency in intensive care patients needing mechanical ventilation. Intensive Care Med 2005;31: 388–92.

[14] Annane D. ICU physicians should abandon the use of etomidate! Intensive Care Med 2005;31: 325–6.

[15] Marik PE, Zaloga GP. Adrenal insufficiency during septic shock. Crit Care Med 2003;31:141–5.

[16] Hoen S, Asehnoune K, Brailly-Tabard S, et al. Costisol response to corticotropin stimulation in trauma patients: influence of hemorrhagic shock. Anesthesiology 2002;97:807–13.

[17] Annane D, Sébille V, Charpentier C, et al. Effect of treatment with low doses of hydrocortisone and fludrocortisone on mortality in patients with septic shock. JAMA 2002;288:862–71.

[18] Loisa P, Uusaro A, Esko R. A single adrenocorticotropic hormone stimulation test does not reveal adrenal insufficiency in septic shock. Anesth Analg 2005;101:1792–8.

[19] Gums JG, Tovar JM. Adrenal gland disorders. In: DiPiro JT, Talbert RT, Yee GC, et al, editors. Pharmacotherapy: a pathophysiologic approach. 6th edition. New York: McGraw-Hill; 2005. p. 1391–406.

[20] Annane D, Bellissant E, Bollaert P-E, et al. Corticosteroids for treating severe sepsis and septic shock. Cochrane Database Syst Rev 2004;1:CD002243.

[21] Oppert M, Schindler R, Husung C, et al. Low-dose hydrocortisone improves shock reversal and reduces cytokine levels in early hyperdynamic septic shock. Crit Care Med 2005;33: 2457–64.

[22] Minneci PC, Deans KJ, Banks SM, et al. Meta-analysis: the effect of steroids on survival and shock during sepsis depends on the dose. Ann Intern Med 2004;141:47–56.

[23] Coursin DB, Wood KE. Corticosteroid supplementation for adrenal insufficiency. JAMA 2002;287:236–40.

[24] Yildiz O, Doganay M, Aygen B, et al. Physiological-dose steroid therapy in sepsis. Crit Care 2002;6:251–8.

[25] Dellinger RP, Carlet JM, Masur H, et al. Surviving sepsis campaign guidelines fro management of severe sepsis and septic shock. Crit Care Med 2004;32:858–73.

[26] Sprung CL. Corticosteroid therapy of septic shock. Available at: Corticus: Clinical Trials. gov. 2005.

[27] Annane D, Cavaillon J-M. Corticosteroids in sepsis: from bench to bedside? Shock 2003; 20:197–207.

[28] De Jonghe B, Sharshar T, Lefaucheur J-P, et al. Paresis acquired in the intensive care unit: a prospective multicenter study. JAMA 2002;288:2859–67.

[29] Confalonieri M, Urbino R, Potena A, et al. Hydrocortisone infusion for severe community-acquired pneumonia. Am J Respir Crit Care Med 2005;171:242–8.

[30] Pizarro CF, Troster EJ, Damiani D, Carcillo JA. Absolute and relative adrenal insufficiency in children with septic shock. Crit Care Med 2005;33:855–9.

[31] Marik PE, Kiminyo K, Zaloga GP. Adrenal insufficiency in critically ill patients with human immunodeficiency virus. Crit Care Med 2002;30:1267–73.

[32] Braams R, Koppeschaar HPF, van de Pavoordt HDWM, van Vroonhoven TJMV. Adrenocortical function in patients with ruptured aneurysm of the abdominal aorta. Intensive Care Med 1998; 24:124–7.

[33] Roberts I, Yates D, Sandercock P, et al. Effect of intravenous corticosteroids on death within 14 days in 10008 adults with clinically significant head injury (MRC CRASH trial): randomised placebo-controlled trial. Lancet 2004;364:1321–8.

[34] Cohan P, Wang C, McArthur DL, et al. Acute secondary adrenal insufficiency after traumatic brain injury: a prospective study. Crit Care Med 2005;33:2358–66.

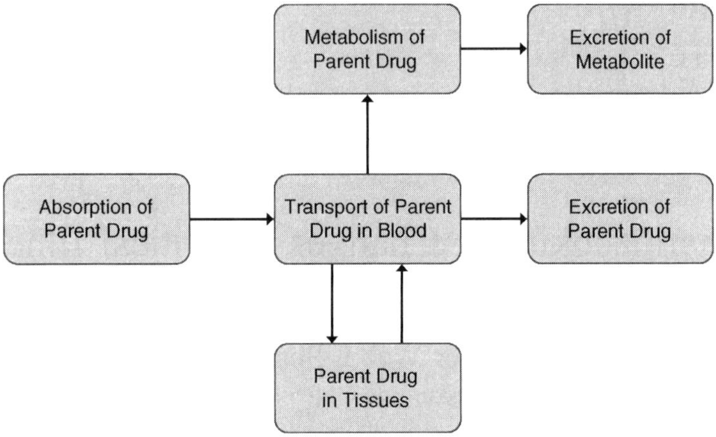

Fig. 1. Simplified pharmacokinetic model of the interrelations between the four basic pharmacokinetic processes of drug absorption, distribution, metabolism, and excretion.

size, solubility, degree of lipophilicity, pKa, and stability are important factors influencing the rate and extent of drug absorption. Environmental characteristics that can affect drug absorption include pH, blood flow, surface area, and gastrointestinal (GI) motility. During critical illness, the delicate balance between the environment within the site of administration and the physical properties of drugs can be significantly different than under normal conditions, resulting in clinically important drug absorption perturbations. These abnormalities may combine with alterations in distribution, metabolism, and elimination to produce less than optimal concentrations at the site of action. Consequently, intravenous administration is the preferred administration route in critically ill patients. Introducing a drug directly into the blood ensures 100% bioavailability by elimination of absorption across membranes and avoidance of first-pass metabolism by the liver. Therefore, when a route other than intravenous is required, the clinician must consider alterations that may impair drug absorption.

Perfusion abnormalities

In shock states, blood flow is directed toward vital organs, such as the brain, heart, and lungs. This redistribution is at the expense of other organs, such as the kidneys and spleen, as well as the GI system. Shunting deprives the periphery of oxygen and nutrients but also reduces the systemic absorption of drugs from the intestines and intramuscular and subcutaneous tissues. This raises concerns about the use of drug delivery routes, such as enteral, transdermal, sublingual, intramuscular, and subcutaneous. An example of this comes from a study that demonstrated significantly reduced anti-Xa concentrations in critically ill patients receiving enoxaparin subcutaneously [2]. Additionally, if there is a need for use of vasoactive agents, the possibility of further reductions in peripheral blood flow must be considered. For a more detailed discussion of specific agents and their effects on regional perfusion abnormalities, the reader is referred to a recent review [3]. Decreased perfusion coupled with high metabolic requirements produces a mismatch that makes the GI system at greater risk for dysfunction and impaired absorption. This dysfunction has been shown to reduce the absorptive capacity of the gut in septic states [4,5]. Although these studies address impaired D-xylose absorption, they also demonstrate the degree of GI dysfunction that could affect drug absorption. Therefore, perfusion abnormalities must be taken into consideration when choosing medication routes in critically ill patients.

Intestinal atrophy

Patients in the intensive care unit (ICU) may undergo varying periods without oral or enteral nutrition. Reasons for this include a clinical decision to withhold enteral feedings because of the patient's hemodynamic status, possible operations, or a patient's intolerance of enteral nutrition. Regardless of the reason for withholding nutrition, it is known that gastrointestinal maintenance and proliferation are primarily stimulated by the presence of food in the gut [6,7]. It has also been shown that starvation results in significant intestinal atrophy [6,8–10], a process that can begin after only 3 days and is not prevented by parenteral nutrition [9,10]. Surface area changes also take place, as evidenced by the decrease in villus height and crypt depth [11]. Dysfunction evident by macroscopic changes of intestinal atrophy is compounded by impaired enzymatic activity on the cellular level [8]. Although investigations directly addressing changes in drug absorption in critically ill patients during periods of starvation are limited, it is likely that cellular dysfunction has the potential to reduce drug absorption from the gut.

Motility dysfunction

Dysmotility of the stomach and small intestine poses an additional concern directly related to early gut hypoperfusion [12]. The required use of narcotics for adequate pain control may further impair GI motility and affect drug absorption [13]. The effect of reduced motility is twofold. First, intolerance of enteral nutrition leads the clinician to abandon the use of the GI tract. Second, if there is an attempt to administer medications enterally, there is sufficient evidence that absorption is altered. Several investigations of delayed gastric emptying focused on acetaminophen kinetics and described a delay in absorption with a diminished peak concentration [14–16]. Heyland and colleagues [14] found no difference in area under the acetaminophen time curve (AUC) for critically ill patients when compared with healthy volunteers, however. Although it is difficult to determine the clinical relevance of these results, for many clinicians, they provide enough doubt to avoid this route until GI function improves.

Physical incompatibilities

Tolerance of enteral nutrition is generally thought to convey the return of GI absorptive function. Physical incompatibilities may still occur, however, despite the appearance of a functioning GI tract. Most drugs are weak acids or bases; as a result, they may exist in the ionized or unionized form. The unionized form is generally more lipophilic and is more likely to be absorbed across the cellular membranes. Therefore, the combination of a drug's pKa and the pH of its surrounding environment can significantly affect absorption by altering its ionized state. The classic example of this is the requirement of an acidic environment for the absorption of itraconazole administered enterally [17]. Stress ulcer prophylaxis using H_2-receptor antagonists or proton-pump inhibitors increases the gastric pH, creating an environment that may alter the lipophilicity of certain drugs similar to that of itraconazole. The risk of pH alterations is continued in the small intestine by the impaired exocrine function of the pancreas, creating a less than optimal environment for drug absorption [18,19].

Another potential problem relates to interactions when a drug is administered concurrently with enteral nutrition. For example, case reports have described a reduction of the prothrombin time (PT) when warfarin was administered with enteral nutrition [20–22]. Prompt prolongation of the PT on discontinuation of enteral nutrition suggests the possibility of warfarin malabsorption secondary to binding to the nutritional formula. An in vitro study measuring the physical interaction between warfarin and an enteral nutrition formula supports these claims [23]. Other drugs with the potential for reduced absorption when given with nutritional formulas include phenytoin [24,25], minocycline [26], and tetracycline [26]. There is mixed evidence concerning such medications as ciprofloxacin [27,28] and fluconazole [29,30], where there seems to be some alterations in absorption but the clinical significance is questioned. Interestingly, there are many drugs for which there are still no data concerning possible interactions with enteral nutrition. This uncertainty further solidifies the use of the intravenous route to ensure 100% bioavailability.

Distribution

Using the most simple pharmacokinetic model, a one-compartment model, distribution of a drug can be mathematically represented by the equation C=D/Vd, where C is the initial concentration of a drug administered as an intravenous bolus, D is the dose, and Vd is the volume of distribution. Distribution of most drugs to the various bodily tissues is dependent on multiple factors, such as blood delivery, degree of protein binding, permeability of the tissues, lipid solubility of the drug, pH of the environment, and pKa of the drug, however. Incorporating these complex interactions requires more intricate pharmacokinetic modeling necessitating the assistance of computers. Surprisingly, a simplified two-compartment model similar to Fig. 1 works well for most drugs. During critical illness, changes occur that can alter factors affecting distribution. To achieve the desired drug concentration, these changes must be considered when determining the dose of certain medications.

pH changes

Frequent changes in pH occur in the critically ill patient as a result of numerous conditions, such as respiratory failure, shock states, and renal failure. As previously mentioned, the pH of the environment affects the ionized state of many drugs. It is well understood that the ionized drug does not penetrate the lipid-based cellular membrane as easily. Therefore, alterations in the ionized state can increase or decrease the extent of distribution of a drug. Because pH changes accompany many other physiologic alterations in critical illness, it is difficult to isolate the degree of impact that pH changes have on distribution. As a result, direct evidence of such effects is limited.

Fluid shifts

Shifts in body fluid have been implicated as a major cause of alterations in distribution. Such physiologic conditions as increased capillary permeability and decreased oncotic pressure seen in septic states provide examples of how potential fluid shifts can occur [31]. The required use of crystalloids or colloids to maintain the intravascular space further drives these shifts [32]. The final result is leakage of large volumes into the interstitium, referred to as "third spacing." Third spacing evident by edema, pleural effusion, and ascites creates a newly expanded compartment into which hydrophilic drugs may be deposited, thus increasing their volume of distribution. Larger than expected volumes of distribution have been well documented in studies of antibiotic administration in critically ill patients [33–38]. This has generally been seen with hydrophilic drugs that have small volumes of distribution, such as the aminoglycosides [34–36,38]. Although these studies have not focused on clinical outcomes, the pharmacokinetic alterations in volume of distribution have the potential to be clinically relevant. This is especially true for such drugs as antibiotics that display concentration-dependent antimicrobial activity. For example, the volume of distribution of gentamicin has been reported to be as large as 0.63 L/kg in critically ill patients [38]. This approached three times that seen in normal individuals and resulted in these patients requiring gentamicin doses as large as 12.4 mg/kg/d to achieve therapeutic concentrations [38]. Fluid shifts alone cannot completely explain observed changes in distribution, however. This is best illustrated by Dasta and Armstrong [34] when they were unable to correlate large cumulative fluid gains with changes in volume of distribution. It is also important to note that several investigators have reported large degrees of variability in volume of distribution resulting in smaller as well as larger than expected values [34,38,39]. This emphasizes the need for the clinician to be cognizant of possible alterations and to monitor drugs with narrow therapeutic indices closely.

Plasma protein binding

Changes in distribution of highly protein-bound drugs are to be expected in the critically ill patient. As is discussed in more detail in the metabolism section of this article, synthesis of such proteins as α_1-acid glycoprotein (AAG) and albumin undergoes significant changes. This results in altered plasma concentrations of these proteins and a corresponding change in the pharmacokinetics of highly protein-bound drugs. The general principle requiring consideration is the fraction of drug that remains unbound. As the concentration of plasma protein decreases, the concentration of protein-bound drug decreases, resulting in an increased unbound fraction. Unbound drug is free to distribute to various tissues in the body, thus increasing the volume of distribution. The reverse is true when the plasma protein concentration increases. The drugs that need to be considered based on protein binding are discussed in the metabolism section of this article.

Metabolism

Hepatic metabolism depends primarily on three physiologic processes: hepatic blood flow (HBF), enzyme activity, and protein binding. Alterations in one or more of these processes result in varying effects on hepatic metabolism depending on the characteristics of the drug. The general equation describing the hepatic clearance of drugs is $CL_H = Q \cdot E$, where CL_H, Q, and E represent total hepatic drug clearance, total HBF, and the hepatic extraction ratio, respectively. The extraction ratio, in turn, is dependent on the drug-metabolizing capabilities of the hepatic enzymes and the protein-binding characteristics of the drug. Specifically, the extraction ratio can be expressed as $E = f_u \cdot CL_{int}/[Q + f_u \cdot CL_{int}]$, where f_u is the unbound fraction of drug and CL_{int} is the intrinsic hepatic clearance or the maximum metabolizing capability of the liver [40]. Extraction ratios can be generally classified as high (>0.7), intermediate (0.3–0.7), and low (<0.3) according to the fraction of drug removed during one pass through the liver. Knowledge of the hepatic extraction ratio for a particular drug is useful in predicting changes in drug metabolism because it relates to changes in HBF, enzyme activity, and protein binding.

Hepatic blood flow

Alterations in HBF can affect drug metabolism by increasing or decreasing drug delivery to the hepatocyte. The most clinically important group of drugs would be those that are highly extracted by the liver (E >0.7). In other words, hepatic metabolism of high hepatic extraction ratio drugs is dependent on HBF and relatively unaltered by changes in hepatic enzyme activity. This occurs because the drug has sufficient time to dissociate from blood components, enter the hepatocyte, and undergo biotransformation or biliary excretion. The efficiency of this process is so great that hepatic perfusion becomes the rate-limiting process in the hepatic metabolism of high extraction. Examples of intermediate- and high-extraction drugs used in the critically ill patient include lidocaine, beta-blockers, morphine, and midazolam.

Sepsis is commonly manifested in critically ill patients and can lead to profound changes in HBF for high-extraction drugs. During the hyperdynamic stage of sepsis, cardiac output (CO) typically increases and blood flow distribution changes to shunt blood flow to vital organs. The opposite is true during late sepsis, where HBF reductions may decrease the clearance of these compounds. Hemorrhagic and other forms of hypovolemic shock, myocardial infarction, and acute heart failure are other problems in critically ill patients in which one can anticipate a decrease in drug clearance for high-extraction drugs. Numerous animal and clinical studies have investigated this phenomenon and have generally confirmed the expected effects of these conditions on HBF, as summarized in a comprehensive review of this topic by McKindley and colleagues [41].

In addition to the effect of critical illness on HBF, iatrogenically induced alterations in HBF may lead to changes in the elimination of intermediate- to high-extraction compounds. Such conditions include the use of mechanical ventilation with or without the administration of positive end-expiratory pressure (PEEP), which is often required in critically ill patients to facilitate delivery of oxygen and gas exchange [42]. Furthermore, drugs may also affect HBF, which could produce significant alterations in the clearance of other drugs whose elimination has blood flow–dependent characteristics. In general, α-adrenoceptor agonists, such as phenylephrine, norepinephrine, epinephrine, and dopamine (>10–12 μg/kg/min), can produce hepatic arterial and portal vein vasoconstriction, leading to decreased total HBF [43]. Vasopressin also has the potential for deceasing HBF [44]. Conversely, nitroglycerin may increase HBF by decreasing portal and hepatic vein resistance. Inotropes like dopamine and dobutamine have been shown to increase HBF by increasing CO. Antihypertensive agents seem to have variable effects on HBF.

Intrinsic clearance

For low-extraction drugs, hepatic clearance is primarily a function of protein binding and intrinsic metabolic activity of the hepatocyte (ie, $CL_H = f_u \cdot CL_{int}$). Slow metabolic enzyme activity, poor diffusion into the hepatocyte, slow dissociation from blood components, and poor biliary transport may all affect the overall CL_H. By far the most important process is metabolic enzyme activity, where induction or suppression of the metabolizing enzymes correspondingly alters the hepatic clearance. Similar to HBF, alterations in CL_H via induction or inhibition of hepatic enzymes can result from physiologic and iatrogenic processes.

Critically ill patients often have significant increases in stress hormones, such as norepinephrine, epinephrine, and cortisol, as well as increases in acute-phase proteins, such AAG and C-reactive protein (CRP). This can occur on admission to an ICU (eg, acute traumatic injury, hemorrhage) or as a complication of critical illness (eg, sepsis). Proinflammatory cytokines (eg, interleukin [IL]-1β, IL-6, tumor necrosis factor-α [TNFα]) have been implicated as important mediators of the physiologic changes observed during the acute-phase response. Given the strong evidence supporting the integral role of cytokines in the etiology of the acute-phase response, in vitro and in vivo investigations into the effect of these proteins on drug metabolism have been conducted. In general, significant inhibition of cytochrome P-450 (CYP450) isoenzymes (phase I metabolism) has been documented [41]. Effects on hepatic phase II conjugative metabolism (eg, glucuronidation, sulfation, acetylation) have also been observed, although the effect is usually less profound than for phase I reactions [41]. Pharmacokinetic studies in critically ill patients in whom this phenomenon has been observed include those using clindamycin [45] and morphine [46].

In contrast to decreased metabolism in acutely stressed patients, metabolism has been demonstrated to increase for selected medications in critically ill patients. One particular subset of critically ill patients that has been evaluated is those with traumatic brain injury (TBI) [47]. Specifically, pentobarbital clearance has been shown to increase over a period of several days, resulting in subtherapeutic concentrations in patients with TBI [48]. Phenytoin clearance has also been shown to be increased during the acute postinjury period after TBI [49,50]. Furthermore, antipyrine, a marker of oxidative metabolism, has been associated with an increased clearance over the study period of 14 days and may indicate that any drug primarily eliminated via oxidative metabolism may be metabolized faster than normal after TBI [50,51]. Phase II enzymatic activity may also be affected in critically ill patients. For example, lorazepam clearance has been shown to increase over a 14-day period in patients with TBI [51]. The increase was not as significant and was delayed when compared with antipyrine metabolism. Similar results have been seen in other critically ill patient subsets (eg, studies of patients with thermal injury studied 3 weeks after injury, where lorazepam clearance was increased nearly fourfold compared with controls, resulting in a significant decrease in the half-life [$t_{1/2}$] from 13.9 to 9.5 hours) [52].

Nutritional supplementation is yet another factor that may affect hepatic drug metabolism. Many critically ill patients are hypermetabolic and exhibit nitrogen wasting after an acute insult. Consequently, early aggressive nutritional intervention is generally recommended, including protein supplementation (15%–20% of caloric intake) in an attempt to attenuate these physiologic alterations and improve patient outcomes. Well-controlled investigations conducted in patients who were not critically ill as well as in normal volunteers using marker substrates have found diet to be an important determinant of drug metabolism [53]. Raising dietary protein intake has generally been associated with an increase in hepatic drug metabolizing capacity [54]. A moderate positive association between phenytoin maximum metabolic velocity (V_{max}) and daily protein intake (range: 0.81–1.88 g/kg/d) was reported in nine patients with severe head injury [50]. The most direct implication of these findings for critically ill patients is to anticipate potential increases in drug clearance concurrent with the aggressive upward titration of protein supplementation over time during their acute management.

Protein binding

Alterations in protein binding primarily affect the hepatic clearance of low-extraction drugs, because high-extraction drugs are completely metabolized independent of protein binding (nonrestrictive hepatic metabolism). In general, hepatic metabolism of low-extraction drugs is restrictive, meaning that metabolism is limited to the unbound fraction. Because only unbound drug is able to diffuse into the hepatocyte, for low-extraction drugs, the fraction unbound correlates with the rate of elimination. The overall importance of alterations in protein binding in the critically ill patient involves the proper interpretation of measured drug concentrations and their pharmacodynamic effect, because only unbound drug is free to interact with its corresponding receptor. Thus, knowledge of the extraction ratio is essential to predicting the pharmacokinetic outcome resulting from protein-binding changes.

It has been demonstrated in critically ill patients that albumin concentrations decrease and AAG synthesis increases during and after traumatic or physiologic stress. This has been demonstrated in multiple critically ill patient subsets. As a result, the pharmacokinetics of albumin-bound or AAG-bound drugs may change. For example, patients with thermal injury demonstrated a two- to threefold increase in AAG concentrations and a twofold decrease in albumin concentrations that lasted the entire 1-month study period [55]. As a result, the fraction unbound increased for acidic drugs primarily bound to albumin (eg, phenytoin, diazepam) but decreased for basic drugs primarily bound to AAG (eg, meperidine, propranolol, lidocaine). This emphasizes the need to monitor the free or unbound concentrations of highly bound drugs in the critically patient. Conversely, the pharmacologic response to drugs highly bound to AAG can be changed dramatically. The unbound fraction of lidocaine decreased from 28% to 15% as AAG concentrations increased in one clinical study. As a result, higher total concentrations of lidocaine were required to achieve pharmacologic effects and were tolerated without toxic effects, because more lidocaine was protein bound and unable to exert pharmacologic effects [56]. Although the overall number of agents for which protein-binding alterations significantly affect drug exposure has been found to be limited based on a recent systematic review, several agents are routinely administered to critically ill patients [57]. In addition to those already addressed, this list includes fentanyl, alfentanil, sufentanil, remifentanil, diltiazem, nicardipine, verapamil, erythromycin, haloperidol, itraconazole, milrinone, and propofol [57].

Excretion

Renal elimination of parent drugs or their metabolites is the primary excretory pathway for most pharmacologic agents regardless of the administration route. This has particular significance in critically ill patients in whom renal dysfunction is commonplace, resulting in decreased renal drug clearance for drugs with extensive renal elimination. In addition, some drugs have active or partially active metabolites that are renally cleared and thus can accumulate in renal dysfunction. Renal dysfunction in critically ill patients can present as preexisting chronic renal failure, new-onset acute renal failure commonly attributable to hypoperfusion or tubular necrosis, or a combination of both. Dosing recommendations for patients with varying degrees of renal dysfunction are widely available from manufacturers' prescribing information, tertiary drug references, and the primary literature. The need for dialysis, the type of dialysis (intermittent versus continuous), and the frequency of dialysis should also be considered. Dosing recommendations for patients requiring dialysis are also available from these sources, albeit with fewer data for newer continuous renal replacement therapies [58]. Thus, the focus of this section is on alterations in renal drug clearance or $t_{1/2}$ in critically ill patients with apparently normal renal function.

The first studies in this area were from the 1970s and investigated aminoglycoside dosing in burn patients in the ICU [59]. It was found that burn patients had more rapid clearance of aminoglycosides than expected. These results, in addition to an increased volume of distribution in these patients, led the authors to promote therapeutic drug monitoring (TDM) and more aggressive dosing of aminoglycosides to achieve serum concentrations that would be expected in patients with normal pharmacokinetic parameters. Since the recognition that burn patients can have increased renal drug clearance, a number of studies have investigated this phenomenon with various drugs and ICU populations. Comparisons in these studies were usually made with historical data in normal volunteers or patients who were not critically ill, although some studies used a concomitant control group. Most studies were performed with antimicrobials. It is especially important to know if a patient population has increased renal clearance of antimicrobials so as to avoid subtherapeutic drug concentrations and treatment failures. These studies are broadly divided into burn, medical and surgical, and trauma patients.

Burn patients

Burn patients have been the most studied subset of critically ill patients relative to renal drug clearance. Such patients are good candidates to have increased renal clearance of drugs because they are hypermetabolic based on nutritional requirements, tend to be young, and are aggressively fluid resuscitated. In reviewing the literature, two trends emerge. First, most studies in burn patients show an increase in mean renal clearance compared with data from normal volunteers or subjects who are not critically ill (Table 1). This is a more pronounced finding than in medical and surgical or trauma patients. Some widely used antimicrobials, such as aminoglycosides, vancomycin, ciprofloxacin, and fluconazole, were found to have increased clearance [59–62]. The data for various β-lactams (eg, extended-spectrum penicillins, cephalosporins, carbapenems) were highly variable, with imipenem being the only agent showing increased

Table 1
Summary of alterations in renal drug clearance in critically ill patients compared with normal subjects or who are not critically ill

Intensive care unit patient population studies	Shorter half-life and/or faster clearance	No change in half-life or clearance	Longer half-life and/or slower clearance
Burn (n = 22)	12	7	3
Medical/surgical (n = 13)	4	6	3
Trauma (n = 7)	2	4	1
All studies (n = 42)	18 (43%)	17 (41%)	7 (17%)

Study drugs include the following agents: aminoglycosides, aztreonam, cefepime, ceftazidime, cimetidine, ciprofloxacin, imipenem, levofloxacin, morphine metabolites, piperacillin, piperacillin/tazobactam, ticarcillin/clavulanic acid, trimethoprim/sulfamethoxazole, and vancomycin.

clearance [63]. Cimetidine and ranitidine were also shown to have increased clearance, which, theoretically, could affect the efficacy of stress ulcer prophylaxis [64,65]. Alternatively, clearance of the glucuronide-6 and -3 metabolites of morphine were found to be within a normal range [66].

The second common trend is that burn patients have a wide degree of variability in renal drug clearance. Thus, even for studies that did not show an overall difference in mean clearance, there are selected patients who have much faster or slower than expected clearance. This is a potentially problematic finding, because drug concentrations that are much more variable than in normal subjects could result in a higher incidence of subtherapeutic or toxic concentrations. Although toxic concentrations in a patient can often be detected by adverse events, the risk of subtherapeutic drug concentrations from rapid clearance is largely undetectable at the bedside and is compounded by the increased volume of distribution commonly seen in these patients.

Medical and surgical patients

The second most frequently studied populations of patients have been grouped for this review as medical and surgical critical care patients (see Table 1). A somewhat different trend was seen in these studies compared with the burn studies. The most common results were no change in renal clearance and an even division between increased and decreased renal clearance (see Table 1). This might be expected, because these patients are less hypermetabolic than burn patients from a nutritional standpoint, are more likely to have lower levels of baseline renal function because of age or preexisting disease, and generally receive less aggressive fluid resuscitation. Because of the nature of these patient populations, there is a high degree of patient heterogeneity. In addition, some studies included patients with active infections, whereas others did not.

Nonetheless, a general result similar to that reported in the burn literature was a high degree of variability in renal clearance within individual studies. Ciprofloxacin and levofloxacin showed more rapid clearance, whereas vancomycin clearance was slower and aminoglycoside clearance was unchanged [67–70]. Similar to the findings in burn patients, renal clearance of β-lactams was highly variable, with imipenem again showing faster clearance [71]. A practical example of the impact of increased renal clearance was seen in a small study that reported subtherapeutic cefepime concentrations in 8 of 10 patients despite an aggressive dose of 2 g [72].

Trauma patients

There are fewer studies in trauma patients than in burn or medical and surgical ICU patients. Trauma patients would seem to be more similar to burn patients than to medical and surgical patients in that they tend to be young and hypermetabolic. Their renal clearance results are actually more similar to the medical and surgical population data, however (see Table 1). Results for β-lactams were again mixed. Ceftazidime had markedly increased clearance, whereas imipenem showed no change and aztreonam had decreased clearance [33,73]. These studies were all from the same investigative group, presumably limiting heterogeneity. Increased trimethoprim and/or sulfamethoxazole clearance was also reported [74]. This is important because of the re-emergence of this agent for treating *Stenotrophomonas maltophilia*. The results for aminoglycosides were mixed; however, one study of once-daily aminoglycoside administration showed that a large percentage of patients had prolonged drug-free intervals because of rapid clearance and may require more intensive TDM [75]. Similar to the burn and medical and surgical ICU patient population literature, there was often a wide degree of variability in clearance within studies.

Dosing and monitoring considerations

Potential alterations in oral, intramuscular, or subcutaneous bioavailability make the intravenous administration route generally preferred in critically ill patients. Enteral administration becomes a viable option when the patient is stabilized and GI system function has returned. Drug-nutrient interactions must always be a consideration, however, and appropriate monitoring should be conducted for drugs with narrow therapeutic indices. Determination of the initial dose must take into consideration the alterations in volume of distribution found in critically ill patients. For example, increases in loading doses are desirable for drugs with exhibited increases in volume of distribution in specific critically ill patient subsets. Generally, decreases in hepatic drug clearance requires a dosage decrease to avoid drug accumulation, whereas increased drug clearance may require a dosage increase to achieve a comparable effect compared with patients with normal clearance. The high degree of variability in renal clearance from studies performed in critically ill patients makes it difficult to extrapolate these data to the bedside. As such, it is imperative that clinicians be familiar with manufacturers' dosing recommendations so as to avoid underdosing or overdosing selected medications having extensive renal elimination. Individualization of dosing through TDM should be used when available (aminoglycosides and vancomycin) for minimization of toxicity and maximization of efficacy.

Summary

It is clear that many physiologic alterations can occur during critical illness, resulting in the potential for significant changes in drug absorption, distribution, metabolism, or excretion. Furthermore, these alterations may not always be static but rather change over time in this dynamic patient subset (Fig. 2). Thus, critical care practitioners must not only be well versed on documented pharmacokinetic changes in the critically ill but be vigilant in their monitoring of these agents. Only then can optimal use of these agents occur in terms of maximizing their efficacy and minimizing adverse events.

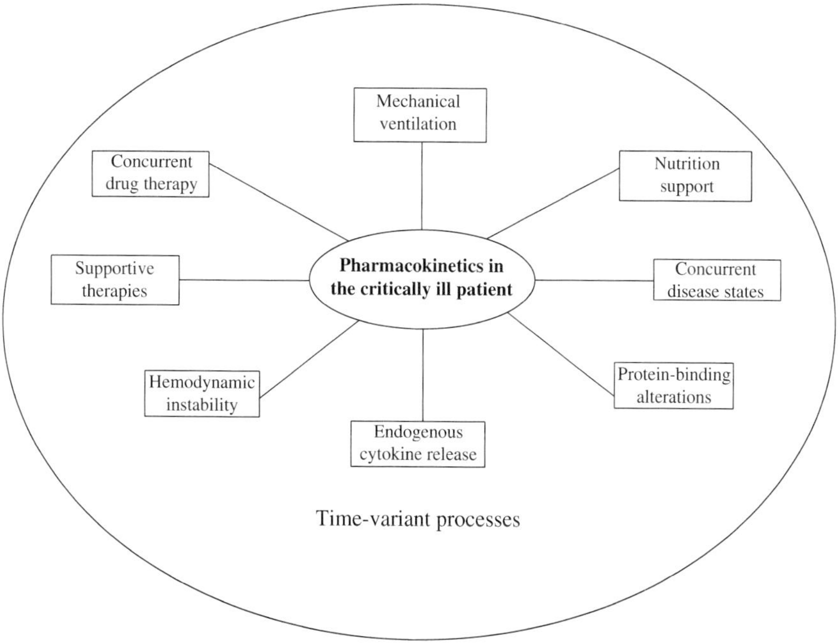

Fig. 2. Potential factors affecting drug disposition in critically ill patients. The possibility of temporal changes in these factors must also be considered secondary to the dynamic nature of this patient subset. (*Modified from* Herfindal ET, Gourley DR. Textbook of therapeutics, drug and disease management. 7th edition. New York: Lippincott Williams & Wilkins; 2000. p. 2079; with permission.)

References

[1] Power BM, Forbes AM, van Heerden PV, et al. Pharmacokinetics of drugs used in critically ill adults. Clin Pharmacokinet 1998;34(1):25–56.

[2] Priglinger U, Delle Karth G, Geppert A, et al. Prophylactic anticoagulation with enoxaparin: is the subcutaneous route appropriate in the critically ill? Crit Care Med 2003;31(5): 1405–9.

[3] Beale RJ, Hollenberg SM, Vincent JL, et al. Vasopressor and inotropic support in septic shock: an evidence-based review. Crit Care Med 2004;32(11 Suppl):S455–65.

[4] Singh G, Chaudry KI, Chudler LC, et al. Sepsis produces early depression of gut absorptive capacity: restoration with diltiazem treatment. Am J Physiol 1992;263(1 Pt 2):R19–23.

[5] Johnston JD, Harvey CJ, Menzies IS, et al. Gastrointestinal permeability and absorptive capacity in sepsis. Crit Care Med 1996;24(7):1144–9.

[6] Ecknauer R, Sircar B, Johnson LR. Effect of dietary bulk on small intestinal morphology and cell renewal in the rat. Gastroenterology 1981;81(4):781–6.

[7] Levine GM, Deren JJ, Yezdimir E. Small-bowel resection. Oral intake is the stimulus for hyperplasia. Am J Dig Dis 1976;21(7):542–6.

[8] Levine GM, Deren JJ, Steiger E, et al. Role of oral intake in maintenance of gut mass and disaccharide activity. Gastroenterology 1974;67(5):975–82.

[9] Hughes CA, Dowling RH. Speed of onset of adaptive mucosal hypoplasia and hypofunction in the intestine of parenterally fed rats. Clin Sci (Lond) 1980;59(5):317–27.

[10] Hernandez G, Velasco N, Wainstein C, et al. Gut mucosal atrophy after a short enteral fasting period in critically ill patients. J Crit Care 1999;14(2):73–7.

[11] Clarke RM. The time-course of changes in mucosal architecture and epithelial cell production and cell shedding in the small intestine of the rat fed after fasting. J Anat 1975;120(Pt 2): 321–7.

[12] Hassoun HT, Kone BC, Mercer DW, et al. Post-injury multiple organ failure: the role of the gut. Shock 2001;15(1):1–10.

[13] Jacobi J, Fraser GL, Coursin DB, et al. Clinical practice guidelines for the sustained use of sedatives and analgesics in the critically ill adult. Crit Care Med 2002;30(1):119–41.

[14] Heyland DK, Tougas G, King D, et al. Impaired gastric emptying in mechanically ventilated, critically ill patients. Intensive Care Med 1996;22(12):1339–44.

[15] MacLaren R, Kuhl DA, Gervasio JM, et al. Sequential single doses of cisapride, erythromycin, and metoclopramide in critically ill patients intolerant to enteral nutrition: a randomized, placebo-controlled, crossover study. Crit Care Med 2000;28(2):438–44.

[16] Heyland DK, Tougas G, Cook DJ, et al. Cisapride improves gastric emptying in mechanically ventilated, critically ill patients. A randomized, double-blind trial. Am J Respir Crit Care Med 1996;154(6 Pt 1):1678–83.

[17] Lim SG, Sawyerr AM, Hudson M, et al. Short report: the absorption of fluconazole and itraconazole under conditions of low intragastric acidity. Aliment Pharmacol Ther 1993;7(3): 317–21.

[18] Tribl B, Sibbald WJ, Vogelsang H, et al. Exocrine pancreatic dysfunction in sepsis. Eur J Clin Invest 2003;33(3):239–43.

[19] Tribl B, Madl C, Mazal PR, et al. Exocrine pancreatic function in critically ill patients: septic shock versus non-septic patients. Crit Care Med 2000;28(5):1393–8.

[20] Howard PA, Hannaman KN. Warfarin resistance linked to enteral nutrition products. J Am Diet Assoc 1985;85(6):713–5.

[21] Penrod LE, Allen JB, Cabacungan LR. Warfarin resistance and enteral feedings: 2 case reports and a supporting in vitro study. Arch Phys Med Rehabil 2001;82(9):1270–3.

[22] Petretich DA. Reversal of osmolite-warfarin interaction by changing warfarin administration time (letter). Clin Pharm 1990;9(2):93.

[23] Kuhn TA, Garnett WR, Wells BK, et al. Recovery of warfarin from an enteral nutrient formula. Am J Hosp Pharm 1989;46(7):1395–9.

[24] Maynard GA, Jones KM, Guidry JR. Phenytoin absorption from tube feedings. Arch Intern Med 1987;147(10):1821.
[25] Sneed RC, Morgan WT. Interference of oral phenytoin absorption by enteral tube feedings. Arch Phys Med Rehabil 1988;69(9):682–4.
[26] Leyden JJ. Absorption of minocycline hydrochloride and tetracycline hydrochloride. Effect of food, milk, and iron. J Am Acad Dermatol 1985;12(2 Pt 1):308–12.
[27] de Marie S, VandenBergh MF, Buijk SL, et al. Bioavailability of ciprofloxacin after multiple enteral and intravenous doses in ICU patients with severe gram-negative intra-abdominal infections. Intensive Care Med 1998;24(4):343–6.
[28] Mimoz O, Binter V, Jacolot A, et al. Pharmacokinetics and absolute bioavailability of ciprofloxacin administered through a nasogastric tube with continuous enteral feeding to critically ill patients. Intensive Care Med 1998;24(10):1047–51.
[29] Rosemurgy AS, Markowsky S, Goode SE, et al. Bioavailability of fluconazole in surgical intensive care unit patients: a study comparing routes of administration. J Trauma 1995;39(3): 445–7.
[30] Nicolau DP, Crowe H, Nightingale CH, et al. Bioavailability of fluconazole administered via a feeding tube in intensive care unit patients. J Antimicrob Chemother 1995;36(2):395–401.
[31] Suzuki A, Ishihara H, Hashiba E, et al. Detection of histamine-induced capillary protein leakage and hypovolaemia by determination of indocyanine green and glucose dilution method in dogs. Intensive Care Med 1999;25(3):304–10.
[32] Balogh Z, McKinley BA, Cocanour CS, et al. Supranormal trauma resuscitation causes more cases of abdominal compartment syndrome. Arch Surg 2003;138(6):637–42 [discussion: 642–3].
[33] Hanes SD, Wood GC, Herring V, et al. Intermittent and continuous ceftazidime infusion for critically ill trauma patients. Am J Surg 2000;179(6):436–40.
[34] Dasta JF, Armstrong DK. Variability in aminoglycoside pharmacokinetics in critically ill surgical patients. Crit Care Med 1988;16(4):327–30.
[35] Ronchera-Oms CL, Tormo C, Ordovas JP, et al. Expanded gentamicin volume of distribution in critically ill adult patients receiving total parenteral nutrition. J Clin Pharm Ther 1995;20(5): 253–8.
[36] Etzel JV, Nafziger AN, Bertino Jr JS. Variation in the pharmacokinetics of gentamicin and tobramycin in patients with pleural effusions and hypoalbuminemia. Antimicrob Agents Chemother 1992;36(3):679–81.
[37] Gous AG, Dance MD, Lipman J, et al. Changes in vancomycin pharmacokinetics in critically ill infants. Anaesth Intensive Care 1995;23(6):678–82.
[38] Zaske DE, Cipolle RJ, Strate RJ. Gentamicin dosage requirements: wide interpatient variations in 242 surgery patients with normal renal function. Surgery 1980;87(2):164–9.
[39] Beckhouse MJ, Whyte IM, Byth PL, et al. Altered aminoglycoside pharmacokinetics in the critically ill. Anaesth Intensive Care 1988;16(4):418–22.
[40] Wilkinson GR, Shand DG. Commentary: a physiological approach to hepatic drug clearance. Clin Pharmacol Ther 1975;18(4):377–90.
[41] McKindley DS, Hanes SD, Boucher BA. Hepatic drug metabolism in critical illness. Pharmacotherapy 1998;18(4):759–78.
[42] Perkins MW, Dasta JF, DeHaven B. Physiologic implications of mechanical ventilation on pharmacokinetics. DICP 1989;23(4):316–23.
[43] Meier-Hellmann A, Reinhart K, Bredle DL, et al. Epinephrine impairs splanchnic perfusion in septic shock. Crit Care Med 1997;25(3):399–404.
[44] Obritsch MD, Bestul DJ, Jung R, et al. The role of vasopressin in vasodilatory septic shock. Pharmacotherapy 2004;24(8):1050–63.
[45] Mann HJ, Townsend RJ, Fuhs DW, et al. Decreased hepatic clearance of clindamycin in critically ill patients with sepsis. Clin Pharm 1987;6(2):154–9.
[46] Macnab MS, Macrae DJ, Guy E, et al. Profound reduction in morphine clearance and liver blood flow in shock. Intensive Care Med 1986;12(5):366–9.
[47] Boucher BA, Hanes SD. Pharmacokinetic alterations after severe head injury. Clinical relevance. Clin Pharmacokinet 1998;35(3):209–21.

[48] Heinemeyer G, Roots I, Dennhardt R. Monitoring of pentobarbital plasma levels in critical care patients suffering from increased intracranial pressure. Ther Drug Monit 1986;8(2): 145–50.
[49] Boucher BA, Rodman JH, Jaresko GS, et al. Phenytoin pharmacokinetics in critically ill trauma patients. Clin Pharmacol Ther 1988;44(6):675–83.
[50] McKindley DS, Boucher BA, Hess MM, et al. Effect of acute phase response on phenytoin metabolism in neurotrauma patients. J Clin Pharmacol 1997;37(2):129–39.
[51] Boucher BA, Kuhl DA, Fabian TC, et al. Effect of neurotrauma on hepatic drug clearance. Clin Pharmacol Ther 1991;50(5 Pt 1):487–97.
[52] Martyn J, Greenblatt DJ. Lorazepam conjugation is unimpaired in burn trauma. Clin Pharmacol Ther 1988;43(3):250–5.
[53] Walter-Sack I, Klotz U. Influence of diet and nutritional status on drug metabolism. Clin Pharmacokinet 1996;31(1):47–64.
[54] Fagan TC, Oexmann MJ. Effects of high protein, high carbohydrate, and high fat diets on laboratory parameters. J Am Coll Nutr 1987;6(4):333–43.
[55] Martyn JA, Abernethy DR, Greenblatt DJ. Plasma protein binding of drugs after severe burn injury. Clin Pharmacol Ther 1984;35(4):535–9.
[56] Edwards DJ, Lalka D, Cerra F, et al. Alpha1-acid glycoprotein concentration and protein binding in trauma. Clin Pharmacol Ther 1982;31(1):62–7.
[57] Benet LZ, Hoener BA. Changes in plasma protein binding have little clinical relevance. Clin Pharmacol Ther 2002;71(3):115–21.
[58] Joy MS, Matzke GR, Armstrong DK, et al. A primer on continuous renal replacement therapy for critically ill patients. Ann Pharmacother 1998;32(3):362–75.
[59] Boucher BA, Kuhl DA, Hickerson WL. Pharmacokinetics of systemically administered antibiotics in patients with thermal injury. Clin Infect Dis 1992;14(2):458–63.
[60] Rybak MJ, Albrecht LM, Berman JR, et al. Vancomycin pharmacokinetics in burn patients and intravenous drug abusers. Antimicrob Agents Chemother 1990;34(5):792–5.
[61] Garrelts JC, Jost G, Kowalsky SF, et al. Ciprofloxacin pharmacokinetics in burn patients. Antimicrob Agents Chemother 1996;40(5):1153–6.
[62] Boucher BA, King SR, Wandschneider HL, et al. Fluconazole pharmacokinetics in burn patients. Antimicrob Agents Chemother 1998;42(4):930–3.
[63] Dailly E, Kergueris MF, Pannier M, et al. Population pharmacokinetics of imipenem in burn patients. Fundam Clin Pharmacol 2003;17(6):645–50.
[64] Ziemniak JA, Watson WA, Saffle JR, et al. Cimetidine kinetics during resuscitation from burn shock. Clin Pharmacol Ther 1984;36(2):228–33.
[65] Martyn JA, Bishop AL, Oliveri MF. Pharmacokinetics and pharmacodynamics of ranitidine after burn injury. Clin Pharmacol Ther 1992;51(4):408–14.
[66] Perreault S, Choiniere M, du Souich PB, et al. Pharmacokinetics of morphine and its glucuronidated metabolites in burn injuries. Ann Pharmacother 2001;35(12):1588–92.
[67] Rebuck JA, Fish DN, Abraham E. Pharmacokinetics of intravenous and oral levofloxacin in critically ill adults in a medical intensive care unit. Pharmacotherapy 2002;22(10):1216–25.
[68] Hassan E, Ober JD. Predicted and measured aminoglycoside pharmacokinetic parameters in critically ill patients. Antimicrob Agents Chemother 1987;31(11):1855–8.
[69] Garaud JJ, Regnier B, Inglebert F, et al. Vancomycin pharmacokinetics in critically ill patients. J Antimicrob Chemother 1984;14(Suppl D):53–7.
[70] Forrest A, Nix DE, Ballow CH, et al. Pharmacodynamics of intravenous ciprofloxacin in seriously ill patients. Antimicrob Agents Chemother 1993;37(5):1073–81.
[71] Tegeder I, Bremer F, Oelkers R, et al. Pharmacokinetics of imipenem-cilastatin in critically ill patients undergoing continuous venovenous hemofiltration. Antimicrob Agents Chemother 1997;41(12):2640–5.
[72] Lipman J, Wallis SC, Rickard C. Low plasma cefepime levels in critically ill septic patients: pharmacokinetic modeling indicates improved troughs with revised dosing. Antimicrob Agents Chemother 1999;43(10):2559–61.

[73] McKindley DS, Boucher BA, Hess MM, et al. Pharmacokinetics of aztreonam and imipenem in critically ill patients with pneumonia. Pharmacotherapy 1996;16(5):924–31.
[74] Hess MM, Boucher BA, Laizure SC, et al. Trimethoprim-sulfamethoxazole pharmacokinetics in trauma patients. Pharmacotherapy 1993;13(6):602–6.
[75] Barletta JF, Johnson SB, Nix DE, et al. Population pharmacokinetics of aminoglycosides in critically ill trauma patients on once-daily regimens. J Trauma 2000;49(5):869–72.

ELSEVIER
SAUNDERS

Crit Care Clin 22 (2006) 273–290

CRITICAL
CARE
CLINICS

Principles and Practices of Medication Safety in the ICU

Sandra Kane-Gill, PharmD, MSc[a,*], Robert J. Weber, MSc[b]

[a]School of Pharmacy, Center for Pharmacoinformatics and Outcomes Research, University of Pittsburgh, 918 Salk Hall, 3501 Terrace Street, Pittsburgh, PA 15261, USA
[b]School of Pharmacy, University of Pittsburgh Medical Center, 200 Lothrop Street, 302 Scaife Hall, Pittsburgh, PA 15213, USA

The 1999 Institute of Medicine report (*To Err is Human*) estimates that more than one million injuries and nearly 100,000 deaths occur annually in the United States as a result of preventable mistakes in health care [1]. All medical mistakes are a significant concern to patients, health care organizations, and clinicians. Among these are medication errors, which occur at a mean rate of 19% in hospitalized adults [2].

The United States Pharmacopeia (USP) MEDMARX voluntary medication error reporting system recently published its 5-year analysis of reported medication errors. More than 235,000 medication errors were reported in 2003 in the United States; at least 2% of those errors resulted in significant patient harm (eg, injury requiring treatment, prolonged hospital stay, death) [3]. This report emphasized the inherent risk in the medication process to cause harm, and served as a "call to action" to develop a systematic approach to patient safety within United States hospitals.

Experts have been critical recently of advances in patient safety. An analysis 5 years after the Institute of Medicine Report cites little or no improvement in outcomes associated with patient safety [4]. This finding indicates that knowledge, intervention, and research in medication patient safety are needed to affect patient care outcomes positively.

The patient care that is provided in ICUs continues to grow in its sophistication because of the introduction of new drugs and technologies. For example,

* Corresponding author.
E-mail address: kanesl@upmc.edu (S. Kane-Gill).

doi:10.1016/j.ccc.2006.02.005 ***criticalcare.theclinics.com***

the US Food and Drug Administration approved 230 drugs for distribution between 1997 and 2003 [5–11]. In 2000, 33 new drug entities were marketed; 10 of these drugs were approved for use in the ICU [8,12]. More than half of these new drugs that are used in the ICU fall into a therapeutic class that is error prone or results in a serious clinical outcome as a result of a medication error, according to the USP MEDMARX report [3]. This illustrates that "high-risk" medications are used often in ICUs.

The inherent characteristics of an ICU and the nature of its patients pose a risk for medication errors. The ICU environment often is fast paced, with frequently changing patient conditions that require rapid decisions for patient care. Nearly two thirds of all patients in the ICU are prescribed multiple intravenous medications, and on average use approximately twice as many medications as do patients who are not in an ICU [13]. As a result, patients in an ICU may be at greater risk for medication errors because of mishaps in communication amongst caregivers, errors in calculating medication dosages, and improper medication administration. For example, intravenous infusions for 71 patients who were admitted to a surgical ICU were reviewed for accuracy in dosage calculation and administered dosage. The researchers observed an error rate of 10.6% (105.9 errors per 1000 patient-days) [14]. Practically applied, these results suggest that 1 in every 10 intravenous infusions in an ICU is prepared or administered in error. Medications that patients in an ICU receive intravenously include anticoagulants, vasoactive medications, and adrenergic stimulants. These potent drugs are associated with adverse drug events (ADEs), even when used properly. The possibility for medication error serves to increase the risk for an ADE occurrence with those medications.

The Institute for Safe Medication Practices, a United States- and Canada-based organization that is committed to reducing medication errors, identifies the ICU as a risk area for such errors because many drugs that are used in those areas are considered "high risk" for errors and ADEs. Despite the known risks and inherent danger of medication errors in ICUs, physicians and other heathcare workers do not believe that their hospital leadership is moving their institutions actively toward becoming safety centered institutions [15]. On average, 62% of healthcare professionals doubt that their concerns about patient safety would be acted upon by management. Further, a similar number (64%) believe that management would never compromise productivity for safety concerns.

This article provides an overview of the practices and principles of medication safety in the ICU and a guide to practical information that critical care clinicians can apply to the care of patients in the ICU. This article describes the importance of medication safety in the ICU by reviewing the prevalence of errors and their impact on patient care. The general principles of medication safety, including defining, identifying, reporting, classifying, and analyzing medication errors, also are reviewed. Finally, a summary of safe medication practices in the ICU is provided, along with practical suggestions to improve medication safety in the ICU.

Medication errors in the ICU: scope of the problem

Prevalence

The prevalence of medication errors in the ICU varies widely; a full review of the literature is summarized in Table 1. For comparison purposes the prevalence rates were changed to number of errors per 1000 patient-days when possible. The frequency of medication errors ranged from 1.2 to 947 per 1000 patient-days with a median of 105.9 per 1000 patient-days in adult ICUs and 24.1 per 1000 patient-days in neonatal/pediatric ICUs [14,16–18]. The large variation in error rates can be attributed to mechanisms of detection, type of ICU, number of ICUs evaluated, existing technology in the ICU, number of institutions evaluated, definition of medication error, and node in the medication use process under investigation. Another variable is the inclusion of more than one error per prescription, which was found in the study with the highest error rate (947 errors per 1000 patient-days) [17]. The low rate of 1.2 errors per 1000 patient-days is likely explained by the reliance of this study on voluntary reporting, which may be lower than at other institutions [16].

Comparing the error rates of the ICU with other units within an institution is helpful in understanding the significance of medication errors in the ICU setting. One study demonstrated that errors occur more commonly in the ICU, with an error rate ratio of 2.17 [19]. The need for assessing ICU medication error frequency is highlighted by the finding that 78% of the serious medical errors that occurred in the ICU were attributed to medications [20].

A definitive study to examine the incidence of medical errors in the ICU was conducted in a medical ICU (MICU) and coronary care unit (CCU) over a 1-year period by researchers at Brigham and Women's Hospital in Boston, Massachusetts. The Critical Care Safety Study's goal was to examine the prevalence and nature of adverse events and serious medical errors in the ICU [20]. Researchers gathered data from four areas: direct observation of care, voluntary reports, computerized ADE monitoring, and chart review. Incidents were reviewed by expert panels and categorized by type and severity of error.

Results of the Critical Care Safety Study show that medications were involved in a large percentage of ADEs, and that 78% of the serious errors involved medications [20]. The overall medication error rate was 12.7% and 12.1% for the MICU and CCU, respectively. Medication error types most frequently involved the wrong dosage of a medication; the most common drugs that were associated with medication errors were cardiovascular drugs (24%), anticoagulants (20%), and anti-infective agents (13%). The researchers indicated their intention to institute system changes after the conclusion of this study. Examples include a new facility that is conducive to organized communication and workflow, "on-line" reporting of incidents, barcode medication administration, house-staff work schedule changes, and infusion pumps that are capable of cross-checking medication orders against the programming function by the nursing staff (eg, "Smart" pumps).

Table 1
Review of published studies on medication errors in the ICU

Reference	Type of ICU	Rate of medication errors[a]	Common error types	Medication process node	Common drugs
[16]	Medical-surgical	1.2 per 1000 patient-days	Not specified	All nodes (voluntary reports)	Not specified
[73]	Neonatal and pediatric	8.8 per 1000 patient-days 14.7 per 100 admissions	Wrong time, wrong rate, wrong dose	All nodes (voluntary reports)	Intralipids/hyperalimentation, anti-infectives, dialysis solution, heparin, labetalol, morphine, nitroprusside
[27]	Neonatal and pediatric	284 in a year	Wrong dose administration	All nodes (voluntary reports)	Anticoagulants, catecholamines, electrolytes
[18]	Neonatal	24.1 per 1000 neonatal activity days	Incorrect dose, incomplete prescriptions	All nodes (voluntary reports)	Mostly parenteral medications, specifically antibiotics
[74]	Cardiac surgery, general ICU	7.6 per 1000 patient-days 36 per 9366 patients	Wrong concentration, wrong medication/infusion	All nodes	Not specified
[75]	Neonatal	47% (581/1230) of medical events were due to medications	Wrong dose and schedule, administration, patient identification	All nodes (voluntary reports)	Not specified
[20]	Coronary and medical	131.5 (CCU) and 127.8 (MICU) per 1000 patient-days	Wrong dose	Prescribing, administering, monitoring	Cardiovascular, anticoagulants, anti-infectives
[76]	Hospitalized patients, including adult and neonatal ICU	4.4 per 1000 patient-days 3.13 per 1000 orders written	Overdose, missing information, underdose	Ordering/prescribing	Antimicrobial, cardiovascular, gastrointestinal
[33]	Pediatric	11.1% of prescriptions evaluated	Missing information, wrong dose, omissions, wrong drug error	Ordering/prescribing	Not specified

[17]	24 ICUs, type not specified	947 per 1000 patient-days 372 per 100 admissions 146 per 1000 new prescriptions	Improperly written, ambiguous, nonstandard nomenclature, written illegibly	Ordering/prescribing	Potassium chloride, heparin, magnesium sulfate, paracetamol, propofol
[77]	Children's hospital, including ICU	32.6 errors per 1000 patient-days (PICU) 8.2 errors per 1000 patient-days (NICU)	Incorrect dosage (overdose and underdose), wrong drug, IV incompatibility	Ordering/prescribing	Antibiotics, theophylline, parenteral nutrition, analgesics, fluid/electrolyte
[51]	Pediatric	30.1 per 100 orders	Missing information, inappropriate dose, wrong units	Ordering/prescribing	Not specified
[19]	Pediatric cardiac ward and ICU	83 per 1000 patient-days 64.7 per 100 admissions	Delayed dose, transcription error, infusion error	Prescribing and administering	Not specified
[78]	Medical	18.1 per 1000 patient-days 6.5 per 100 patient admissions	Delays or omission of prescribed drug, administration of nonprescribed drugs, wrong administration	Prescribing and administering	Not specified
[14]	Surgical	105.9 per 1000 patient-days	Charting inconsistencies	Administering	Dopamine, dobutamine, propofol, cisatracurium, pancuronium, vecuronium, nitroprusside
[24]	Not specified	44.6% (104 of 233 observations)	Wrong time, wrong administration technique, wrong does preparation	Administering	Not specified

(continued on next page)

Table 1 (*continued*)

Reference	Type of ICU	Rate of medication errors[a]	Common error types	Medication process node	Common drugs
[23]	Mixed adult	3.3% (187 errors per 5774 administration observations)	Wrong infusion rate	Administering	Digoxin, lorazepam, heparin, epinephrine
[22]	Medical	6.6% (132 errors per 2009 administration observations)	Physiochemical incompatibility, dosage error	Preparing and administering	Total parenteral nutrition, anti-infectives, bicarbonate solution, bumetanide, almitirine, valproic acid
[79]	Pediatric	38% (81 of the 213 doses administered)	Wrong time of administration, omitted dose	Administering	Anti-infective agents, spasmolytic agents
[80]	Pediatric	26.9% (74 of the 275 administered)	Wrong time, wrong administration technique, preparation errors	Preparing and administering	Furosemide, dobutamine, dopamine, morphine

Abbreviations: IV, intravenous; NICU, neonatal ICU; PICU, pediatric ICU.

[a] Rate of errors was converted to 1000 patient-days if possible.

Medication errors in the ICU occur at various stages of the medication use process, but most occur with drug administration [21]. Because intravenously administered medications are prescribed more commonly in the ICU, this article highlights some studies that evaluated the issue of drug administration to better understand medication errors that are unique to the critically ill population. Causes of errors in medication administration are multifactorial, and a systems approach is necessary to remedy unsafe situations. Investigators from France observed medication administration in an ICU. They observed a 6.6% medication administration error rate, which mostly involved the administration of the wrong dosage of a medication. The study noted errors in preparation technique, compatibilities with other intravenous solutions, and administration technique. The results of the study revealed system issues that were related to the medication process, including interrupted workflow of medication administration, global pharmacy distribution problems, and lack of knowledge on medication preparation by the nursing staff. The study findings led to changes in pharmacy services (placing a pharmacist in the ICU), and a strategy for standardizing medication preparation and dispensing [22]. Repeating the same methods as Tissot and colleagues [22], a study that was performed in ICUs in the United States reported a medication administration error rate of 3.3%; however, all participating ICUs had a physician-led multidisciplinary team that included pharmacists [23].

A Dutch study used a passive observer to determine the frequency and causes of drug administration errors in the ICUs of two hospitals. A 33% error rate was observed, with wrong administration technique as the leading type of error. The investigators determined that the systems for operating the ICUs made a difference in the rate of errors. The ICU with full-time intensive care physicians and approved pharmacy protocols for drug administration had fewer errors (21.5% versus 70.2%). This factor and other system issues, such as staffing on certain days (errors were observed more frequently on a Monday) and lack of familiarity with nursing protocols on nasogastric administration of medication, were suggested as interventions to improve medication safety [24].

Principles of medication safety

The medication process

The medication use process has been categorized into several pivotal nodes (or functions), including ordering/prescribing, transcribing/documenting, dispensing, administering, and monitoring [3,21,25,26]. Evaluating the medication use process by incorporating these nodes allows for a systematic analysis. For example, information may be used to identify the node with the most errors and areas of opportunity for improvement. The prescribing and administration nodes are associated with the most errors based on published data of hospitalized patients [18,21,27]. Each node of the medication use process has the potential for different types of errors. The ordering and administration node errors are associated commonly with lack of drug knowledge and lack of patient information as opposed to the dispensing node, in which errors are caused by failure in drug identity checking and stocking/delivery problems [21]. To develop a better understanding of the nodes that are affected by medication errors in the ICU, the information concerning nodes that was obtained from the literature is reported (see Table 1). The errors that are associated with the administration node have been studied the most in the critically ill population. Error types for the administration node were wrong infusion rate, dose error, wrong time of administration, omitted dose, and physiochemical incompatibilities. Incorporating medication use process nodes in evaluation is a valuable mechanism for the methodical analysis of the source of medication errors, and should be considered for inclusion in future studies that are performed in the ICU.

Table 2
Definitions of medication errors

Reference	Term	Definition
[32,80]	Medication error	Any preventable event that may cause or lead to inappropriate medication use or patient harm while the medication is in the control of the health care professional, patient, or consumer
[20]	Medical error (including medications)	Failure of a planned action to be completed as intended or the use of a wrong plan to achieve an aim
[33]	Medication error	This includes any error, large or small, at any point in the medication system from the time the drug is ordered until the patient receives it
[74]	Error (including medications)	All events when treatment or observation differed from a planned one, and when this was not a part of the natural course of the disease
[19]	Medication error	A mistake made at any stage in the provision of a pharmaceutical product to a patient
[76]	Medication error	Medication orders for the wrong drug, inappropriate frequency, inappropriate dosage form, inappropriate route, inappropriate indication, ordering of unnecessary duplicate/redundant therapy, contraindicated therapy, medications to which the patient was allergic, orders for the wrong patient, or orders missing information required for the dispensing and administration of the drug
[56]	Medication error	Any preventable event that may cause or lead to inappropriate medication use or patient harm while the medication is in the control of the health care professional, patient, or consumer. Such events may be related to professional practice, health care products, procedures, and systems, including prescribing; order communication; product labeling, packaging, and nomenclature; compounding; dispensing; distribution; administration; education; monitoring; and use.
[50]	Medication error	Prescribing decision or prescription writing process resulted in an unintentional significant reduction in the probability of treatment being timely and effective or an unintentional significant increase in the risk of harm when compared with generally accepted practice.

Medication error definitions

As with most definitions in the area of patient safety, a variety of definitions for medication errors exists in the literature. Table 2 lists the definitions that were used in articles discussed within this manuscript. The common theme among these definitions is the classification of a medication error as a preventable mistake, failure, or deviation in planned action that results from inappropriate medication use at any point in the medication use process. The variety of definitions that is used between studies and in different institutions makes benchmarking and comparing data difficult. It is important for the medical community to adopt uniform definitions, and it is reasonable for the ICU and general hospital wards to use the same definitions.

Relationship between medication errors and adverse drug events

The importance of tracking medication errors is emphasized by the potential for the medication error to result in injury referred to as an ADE. The relationship between medication errors and ADEs has been described in the literature [28–32]. It is clear from this literature that a medication error may or may not result in an ADE, and that medication errors are more common than are ADEs. A study by Rothschild and colleagues [20] that was performed in the coronary and medical ICU demonstrated that 129.5 medication errors occurred per 1000 patient-days and resulted in 37.6 ADEs per 1000 patient-days. Another study in the pediatric ICU showed that approximately 1% (16/1335) of prescription errors resulted in ADEs [33]. Various instruments can be helpful in determining if the medication error resulted in an adverse drug reaction [34–38]. Although not all medication errors result in injury, the concern for compromising patient safety is substantial enough to warrant diligent monitoring.

Identification, reporting, and analysis of medication errors

Methods of medication error detection

Submission of a voluntary or solicited incident report is the most common method of detecting medication errors. The characteristics of an effective voluntary reporting system are anonymity, ease of use, and ability to generate information to determine the cause of errors. These characteristics are shared by the Institute for Safe Medication Practices Medication Error Reporting Program and The USP MEDMARX system [39].

The second method of detecting medication administration errors is through direct observation of the medication process [2,22,23]. In this process, a trained observer documents the medications that are administered to a patient by noting the drug, dose, route, and time administered. This observation is compared with the original physician's order, and a medication error is defined as any discrepancy between the actual drug administration and the physician's order. Although this method detects errors in administration only, it creates an awareness of medication administration accuracy.

The third method of detecting medication errors is through direct chart/medical administration record review. This method involves reviewing the medication orders in a patient chart to determine medication errors related to prescribing. This method involves a review of multiple factors that impact medication prescribing, including laboratory values and patient response, among others. This method is resource intensive and requires the development of predetermined criteria for analyzing medication prescribing.

Methods of medication error reporting

MEDMARX offers a comprehensive data collection form for medication errors that includes categorization of error, cause and outcome, and several other useful evaluation components [3]. Although this is an ideal form for reporting errors, it may be too time consuming for the bedside clinician to complete based on the acuity of the patient in the ICU and the need for continuous monitoring. A reasonable alternative is to have the bedside clinician document the location, type of error, and medication step involved, and submit this information as a critical incident report that is investigated by additional personnel. The remaining information, including the root cause and seriousness of the outcome, is determined upon further investigation.

These surveillance programs should indicate the location (ICU versus general ward) of the error or event so that appropriate changes can be initiated based on the patient population; unfortunately, the location often is not documented [40].

Analysis of errors for causes and outcomes

It is necessary to evaluate identified medications errors for root causes and seriousness of outcomes, so that system improvements in patient safety can be made [41]. Because medication errors are common it is important to understand the criteria for prioritizing patient safety efforts within an institution. One criterion for evaluation is the severity [42]. Severity scales exist to aid in this process by assessing the seriousness of the error, the seriousness of the outcome, or both. The scales that have been used in the ICU are described in Table 3. Based on simplicity and clarity, the authors recommend the severity scales that were proposed by Duwe and colleagues [42] or Cimino and colleagues [33]. (For the scale that was developed by Cimino and colleagues the inconsistent 0.5 scores suggests a weighting system that seems to be unnecessary.) Evaluating the cause of the medication error is simpler than severity because the MEDMARX form

Table 3
Error assessment tools

Reference	Assessment	Levels	Instrument description
[18]	Seriousness of error	3 categories (major to minor)	Minor, potential harm, or high risk of harm
[77]	Seriousness of error	3 categories	Significant to potentially lethal
[81]	Seriousness of error	5-point scale	Not critical to very critical
[74]	Seriousness of error	11-point visual analogue scale	No error to most serious error imaginable
[82]	Seriousness of error	11-point visual analogue scale	No potential effect on the patient to an incident that would result in death
[25,56]	Categories of error	9 categories	Types of errors described
[33]	Seriousness of outcome	11-point scale including 0.5 points	No error occurred to death
[19,83]	Seriousness of outcome	7-point scale	Error prevented to error results in death
[74]	Seriousness of outcome	6-point scale	No change to patient died
[42]	Seriousness of outcome	5-point scale	Near miss to catastrophic event
[27]	Seriousness of outcome	3 categories (mild to major)	No intervention required to need for therapeutic intervention specific to the ICU
[50]	Seriousness of outcome	3 categories (mild to major)	No harm to permanent harm or death
[19,83]	Categories of outcome	5 outcomes	Types of outcome described
[3,25]	Categories of patient care	22 levels of patient care	Types of patient care described
[78]	Harm scale	5 categories for error and 5 for level of patient care	Risky situation to death (error) Life-sustaining treatment to care not affected (patient care)

provides a comprehensive list of potential causes that can be used for assessment [3]. Understanding the cause and impact of the event is an essential part of the evaluation process, and the use of an assessment tool provides consistency.

Safe medication practices in the ICU

Intensive surveillance programs

Intensive surveillance programs that include methods of identification, such as voluntary reporting, solicitation of error information from persons involved in the medication use process, direct observation, and chart/medication administration record review, are an optimal approach to error identification because these methods uncover different types of errors [43]. Voluntary reporting alone usually does not yield an optimal rate of reporting. Implementing "no blame" policies, incentive programs, and continuous reminders may improve these efforts. Voluntary reporting also may be increased by providing feedback to staff so they know that their reports make a difference in system-based changes. Although it is recognized that an all-inclusive program that includes chart review is resource intensive and may not be practical, institutions should attempt to optimize the voluntary reporting system. Studies have shown that information obtained from voluntary reporting is of value for system-based changes in the ICU [27,40].

Technology for the prevention of medication errors

Several technologies are being developed to improve patient safety in the ICU. These options include advanced infusion pumps, rule-based decision software, patient simulation for education, telemedicine, bar-code medication administration, and sedation monitoring tools [44–49]. Although the inclusion of computer systems is expensive, implementation of programs, such as computer-based prescriber order entry (CPOE), reduces medication errors in the ICU. Shulman and colleagues [50] reported error rates of 6.7% (69 errors/1036 prescriptions) and 4.8% (117 errors/2429 prescriptions) for hand-written prescriptions and CPOE, respectively ($P < .04$). In a pediatric ICU the medication prescribing errors were reduced by 99% with the implementation of CPOE [51].

A quality control measure for improving medication safety in the ICU is bar-code medication administration, which uses software to compare a bar-coded medication with a patient's .electronic order and other medical information. A nurse is notified when the potential for a medication administration error is detected. This technology reduced medication administration errors by at least 60% [52]. Another technologic advancement is intravenous pumps that use software to check the device programming by the nurse (eg, setting the concentration of the solution and the rate of administration for a medication). These "smart pumps," which are in early clinical testing, seem promising in reduce administration errors, provided the technology is used properly by the end users [44].

Although technologic advancements have the potential to improve patient safety, recognizing their limitations will prevent alternate problems. Process measures should be evaluated subsequent to implementation so that potential problems can be identified [53–55]. A summary of safe medication practices for the ICU is listed in Box 1.

Quality controls in the medication process

A foundational component of improving mediation safety in the ICU is to establish quality controls within the medication process. The first quality control includes proper storage and security of drugs that are prone to medication errors and adverse events by minimizing ICU floor stock. For example, the concentrated electrolyte solution of potassium chloride, 40 mEq, has been administered

Box 1. Safe practice recommendations for the ICU

- Optimize the rate of voluntary reporting using incentive programs and no blame policies. This information can be used to make changes in the medication use process.
- Develop a quality assurance program that periodically uses direct observation for evaluation of medication errors.
- Implement technological advancements (CPOE, bar-coding, advanced infusion pumps) that reduce medication errors but have an ongoing quality assessment program that ensures improvement in process and outcome measures.
- Develop standardized intravenous medication preparation and administration policies.
- Implement pharmacy satellite services.
- Develop policy and procedures that control storage and distribution of concentrated electrolyte solutions and emergency medications.
- Implement a medication reconciliation process.
- Use reliable and valid subjective assessment tools to avoid over- and undersedation.
- Use evidence-based medicine to develop guidelines and protocols.
- Have an intensivist-led multidisciplinary team involved in patient care.

mistakenly for furosemide, 40 mg, by direct intravenous injection, which resulted in fatal consequences [56]. Prohibiting the storage of the concentrated potassium chloride medication vial in the ICU floor stock reduces the chance of mistaken use by the patient care staff, which prevents a potentially serious error. In addition, providing organizational standards for the contents of emergency medication carts prevents confusion and potential errors during emergency treatment situations. Establishing a pharmacy satellite service that is staffed by pharmacists and pharmacy technicians also improves safety by minimizing medication floor stock, while reducing the processing time for medication orders. In addition, the pharmacy satellite provides a drug information and clinical resource that is available to clinicians in a more accessible location.

Medication reconciliation is a process that matches the patient's current hospital medication regimen against all medication orders for that patient to prevent drug duplications, inadvertent continuation of discontinued medications, and unnecessary medications. This is particularly important in preventing unnecessary or dangerous medications from being administered when patients are transferred from an ICU to another hospital unit [57]. Using a subjective scale for sedation management can help to prevent errors in dose and duration of sedative agents [58,59].

Evidence-based prescribing programs

Another approach to promote patient safety and prevent medication errors is the development and implementation of evidence-based protocols. Several protocols have been used in the ICU with successful outcomes, including sedation and analgesia [60–62], nutrition [63], dialysis solutions [64], thrombolytic administration [65], thromboprophylaxis [66], and stress ulcer prophylaxis [67]. Also, incorporating critical care bundles into practice also supports positive patient outcomes [68,69]. The University of Pittsburgh Medical Center demonstrated that a drug-use and disease-state management program can be useful for developing multidisciplinary, evidence-based guidelines for standardizing pharmacotherapy in disease management [12].

Multidisciplinary patient care team in the ICU

The use of a physician-led multidisciplinary team for the care of critically ill patients can improve patient safety and clinical outcomes [70,71]. Several reports in the literature confirm this observation. An ICU with full-time intensive care physicians and approved pharmacy protocols for drug administration had fewer errors than did comparators without these measures (21.5% versus 70.2%) [24]. The inclusion of a pharmacist in adult patient care rounds resulted in a 66% reduction in ADEs [72]. The implementation of a pharmacist-led education program in a pediatric ICU resulted in a significant reduction in medication errors [18]. Although there is a cost associated with the salaries for these team members, the reduction in ADEs/medication errors and the ability to create a safer patient environment could result in a positive return on the investment.

Summary

Medication errors occur frequently in the ICU and can result in patient harm. Many medication errors are preventable, and steps can be taken to reduce their frequency. Intensive surveillance programs should exist at every institution to identify, report, and analyze medication errors. A better understanding of the potential risks and common sources of medication errors can contribute to developing systems for their prevention in the ICU. There is a need to use common definitions so that error rates can be compared between units and institutions. This will allow a better understanding of study results, and facilitate the development of safe medication practices that are applicable to all institutions. The implementation of safe medication practices in the ICU reduces medication errors and improves patient outcomes.

References

[1] Kohn LT. The Institute of Medicine report on medical error: overview and implications for pharmacy. Am J Health Syst Pharm 2001;58(1):63–6.

[2] Barker KN, Flynn EA, Pepper GA, et al. Medication errors observed in 36 health care facilities. Arch Intern Med 2002;162(16):1897–903.

[3] Hicks RW, Santell JP, Cousins DD, et al. MEDMARX 5th anniversary data report: a chartbook of 2003 findings and trends, 1999–2003. Rockville, MD: USP Center for the Advancement of Patient Safety; 2004.

[4] Leape LL, Berwick DM. Five years after To Err Is Human: what have we learned? JAMA 2005; 293(19):2384–90.

[5] Hussar DA. New drugs of 2003. J Am Pharm Assoc 2004;44(2):168–206.

[6] Hussar DA. New drugs of 2002. J Am Pharm Assoc 2003;43(2).207–45.

[7] Hussar DA. New drugs of 2001. J Am Pharm Assoc 2002;42(2):227–63.

[8] Hussar DA. New drugs of 2000. J Am Pharm Assoc 2001;41(2):229–72.

[9] Hussar DA. New drugs of 1999. J Am Pharm Assoc 2000;40(2):181–221.

[10] Hussar DA. New drugs of 1998. J Am Pharm Assoc 1999;39(2):151–206.

[11] Hussar DA. New drugs of 1997. J Am Pharm Assoc 1998;38(2):155–95.

[12] Weber RJ, Kane SL, Oriolo VA, et al. Impact of intensive care unit (ICU) drug use on hospital costs: a descriptive analysis, with recommendations for optimizing ICU pharmacotherapy. Crit Care Med 2003;31(1 Suppl):S17–24.

[13] Cullen DJ, Sweitzer BJ, Bates DW, et al. Preventable adverse drug events in hospitalized patients: a comparative study of intensive care and general care units. Crit Care Med 1997;25(8): 1289–97.

[14] Herout PM, Erstad BL. Medication errors involving continuously infused medications in a surgical intensive care unit. Crit Care Med 2004;32(2):428–32.

[15] Pronovost PJ, Weast B, Holzmueller CG, et al. Evaluation of the culture of safety: survey of clinicians and managers in an academic medical center. Qual Saf Health Care 2003;12(6): 405–10.

[16] Abramson NS, Wald KS, Grenvik AN, et al. Adverse occurrences in intensive care units. JAMA 1980;244(14):1582–4.

[17] Ridley SA, Booth SA, Thompson CM. Intensive Care Society's Working Group on Adverse Incident. Prescription errors in UK critical care units. Anaesthesia 2004;59(12):1193–200.

[18] Simpson JH, Lynch R, Grant J, et al. Reducing medication errors in the neonatal intensive care unit. Arch Dis Child Fetal Neonatal Ed 2004;89(6):F480–2.

[19] Wilson DG, McArtney RG, Newcombe RG, et al. Medication errors in paediatric practice: insights from a continuous quality improvement approach. Eur J Pediatr 1998;157(9):769–74.

[20] Rothschild JM, Landrigan CP, Cronin JW, et al. The Critical Care Safety Study: the incidence and nature of adverse events and serious medical errors in intensive care. Crit Care Med 2005; 33(8):1694–700.

[21] Leape LL, Bates DW, Cullen DJ, et al. Systems analysis of adverse drug events. ADE Prevention Study Group. JAMA 1995;274(1):35–43.

[22] Tissot E, Cornette C, Demoly P, et al. Medication errors at the administration stage in an intensive care unit. Intensive Care Med 1999;25(4):353–9.

[23] Calabrese AD, Erstad BL, Brandl K, et al. Medication administration errors in adult patients in the ICU. Intensive Care Med 2001;27(10):1592–8.

[24] van den Bemt PM, Fijn R, van der Voort PH, et al. Frequency and determinants of drug administration errors in the intensive care unit. Crit Care Med 2002;30(4):846–50.

[25] Brown MM. Managing medication errors by design. Crit Care Nurs Q 2001;24(3):77–97.

[26] Nadzam DM. Development of medication-use indicators by the Joint Commission on Accreditation of Healthcare Organizations. Am J Hosp Pharm 1991;48(9):1925–30.

[27] Frey B, Buettiker V, Hug MI, et al. Does critical incident reporting contribute to medication error prevention? Eur J Pediatr 2002;161(11):594–9.

[28] Bates DW, Boyle DL, Vander Vliet MB, et al. Relationship between medication errors and adverse drug events. J Gen Intern Med 1995;10(4):199–205.
[29] Nebeker JR, Barach P, Samore MH. Clarifying adverse drug events: a clinician's guide to terminology, documentation, and reporting. Ann Intern Med 2004;140(10):795–801.
[30] Morimoto T, Gandhi TK, Seger AC, et al. Adverse drug events and medication errors: detection and classification methods. Qual Saf Health Care 2004;13(4):306–14.
[31] Kane-Gill SL, Dasta JF, Schneider PJ, et al. Monitoring abnormal laboratory values as antecedents to drug induced injury. Journal of Trauma-Injury Infection and Critical Care 2005;59: 1457–62.
[32] Anonymous. Suggested definitions and relationships among medication misadventures, medication errors, adverse drug events, and adverse drug reactions. Am J Health Syst Pharm 1998;55(2):165–6.
[33] Cimino MA, Kirschbaum MS, Brodsky L, et al. Child Health Accountability I. Assessing medication prescribing errors in pediatric intensive care units. Pediatr Crit Care Med 2004;5(2): 124–32.
[34] Kramer MS, Leventhal JM, Hutchinson TA, et al. An algorithm for the operational assessment of adverse drug reactions. I. Background, description, and instructions for use. JAMA 1979; 242(7):623–32.
[35] Karch FE, Lasagna L. Toward the operational identification of adverse drug reactions. Clin Pharm Ther 1977;21(3):247–54.
[36] Naranjo CA, Busto U, Sellers EM, et al. A method for estimating the probability of adverse drug reactions. Clin Pharm Ther 1981;30(2):239–45.
[37] Kane-Gill SL, Kirisci L, Pathak DS. Are the Naranjo criteria reliable and valid for determination of adverse drug reactions in the intensive care unit? Ann Pharmacother 2005;39(11): 1823–7.
[38] Jones JK. Definition of events associated with drugs: regulatory perspectives. J Rheumatol Suppl 1988;17:14–9.
[39] Leape LL. Reporting of adverse events. N Engl J Med 2002;347(20):1633–8.
[40] Kane-Gill SL, Devlin JW. Adverse drug event reporting in the intensive care unit: a survey of current practices. Ann Pharmacother 2006; in press.
[41] Schneider PJ, Hartwig SC. Use of severity-indexed medication error reports to improve quality. Hospital Pharmacy 1994;29(3):205–6.
[42] Duwe B, Fuchs BD, Hansen-Flaschen J. Failure mode and effects analysis application to critical care medicine. Crit Care Clin 2005;21(1):21–30.
[43] Jha AK, Kuperman GJ, Teich JM, et al. Identifying adverse drug events: development of a computer-based monitor and comparison with chart review and stimulated voluntary report. J Am Med Inform Assoc 1998;5(3):305–14.
[44] Rothschild JM, Keohane CA, Cook EF, et al. A controlled trial of smart infusion pumps to improve medication safety in critically ill patients. Crit Care Med 2005;33(3):533–40.
[45] Patow CA. Improving patient safety through simulation technology. AHIP Cover 2004;45(3): 74–7.
[46] Breslow MJ, Rosenfeld BA, Doerfler M, et al. Effect of a multiple-site intensive care unit telemedicine program on clinical and economic outcomes: an alternative paradigm for intensivist staffing. Crit Care Med 2004;32(1):31–8 [erratum appears in Crit Care Med 2004;32(7):1632].
[47] Zarowitz BJ, Petitta A, Rudis MI, et al. Bar code documentation of pharmacotherapy services in intensive care units. Pharmacotherapy 1996;16(2):261–6.
[48] Zarowitz BJ, Petitta A, Mlynarek M, et al. Bar-code technology applied to drug-use evaluation. Am J Hosp Pharm 1993;50(5):935–9.
[49] Olson DM, Cheek DJ, Morgenlander JC. The impact of bispectral index monitoring on rates of propofol administration. AACN Clin Issues 2004;15(1):63–73.
[50] Shulman R, Singer M, Goldstone J, et al. Medication errors: a prospective cohort study of hand-written and computerised physician order entry in the intensive care unit. Crit Care 2005; 9(5):R516–21.

[51] Potts AL, Barr FE, Gregory DF, et al. Computerized physician order entry and medication errors in a pediatric critical care unit. Pediatrics 2004;113(1 Pt 1):59–63.
[52] Cummings J, Bush P, Smith D, et al. UHC Bar Coding Task Force. Bar-coding medication administration overview and consensus recommendations. Am J Health Syst Pharm 2005;62(24): 2626–30.
[53] Ali NA, Mekhjian HS, Kuehn PL, et al. Specificity of computerized physician order entry has a significant effect on the efficiency of workflow for critically ill patients. Crit Care Med 2005; 33(1):110–4.
[54] Koppel R, Metlay JP, Cohen A, et al. Role of computerized physician order entry systems in facilitating medication errors. JAMA 2005;293(10):1197–203.
[55] Han YY, Carcillo JA, Venkataraman ST, et al. Unexpected increased mortality after implementation of a commercially sold computerized physician order entry system. Pediatrics 2005;116(6):1506–12.
[56] National Coordinating Council for Medication Error Reporting and Prevention. What is a medication error? Available at: http://www.nccmerp.org/aboutMedErrors.html. Accessed January 4, 2006.
[57] Pronovost P, Weast B, Schwarz M, et al. Medication reconciliation: a practical tool to reduce the risk of medication errors. J Crit Care 2003;18(4):201–5.
[58] Devlin JW, Fraser GL, Kanji S, et al. Sedation assessment in critically ill adults. Ann Pharmacother 2001;35(12):1624–32.
[59] Watson BD, Kane-Gill SL. Sedation assessment in critically ill adults: 2001–2004 update. Ann Pharmacother 2004;38(11):1898–906.
[60] MacLaren R, Plamondon JM, Ramsay KB, et al. A prospective evaluation of empiric versus protocol-based sedation and analgesia. Pharmacotherapy 2000;20(6):662–72.
[61] Devlin JW, Holbrook AM, Fuller HD. The effect of ICU sedation guidelines and pharmacist interventions on clinical outcomes and drug cost. Ann Pharmacother 1997;31(6):689–95.
[62] Hynes-Gay P, Leo M, Molino-Carmona S, et al. Optimizing sedation and analgesia in mechanically ventilated patients—an evidence-based approach. Dynamics 2003;14(4):10–3.
[63] Mackenzie SL, Zygun DA, Whitmore BL, et al. Implementation of a nutrition support protocol increases the proportion of mechanically ventilated patients reaching enteral nutrition targets in the adult intensive care unit. JPEN J Parenter Enteral Nutr 2005;29(2):74–80 [erratum appears in JPEN J Parenter Enteral Nutr. 2005;29(4):xii].
[64] Paganini EP, Sandy D, Moreno L, et al. The effect of sodium and ultrafiltration modelling on plasma volume changes and haemodynamic stability in intensive care patients receiving haemodialysis for acute renal failure: a prospective, stratified, randomized, cross-over study. Nephrol Dial Transplant 1996;11(Suppl 8):32–7.
[65] Kynman G. Thrombolysis: the development of unit guidelines. Intensive Crit Care Nurs 1997; 13(1):30–41.
[66] Misra M, Roitberg B, Ebersole K, et al. Prevention of pulmonary embolism by combined modalities of thromboprophylaxis and intensive surveillance protocol. Neurosurgery 2004;54(5): 1099–102 [discussion 1102–3].
[67] Hatton J, Lu WY, Rhoney DH, et al. A step-wise protocol for stress ulcer prophylaxis in the neurosurgical intensive care unit. Surg Neurol 1996;46(5):493–9.
[68] Vincent JL. Give your patient a fast hug (at least) once a day. Crit Care Med 2005;33(6):1225–9.
[69] Crunden E, Boyce C, Woodman H, et al. An evaluation of the impact of the ventilator care bundle. Nurs Crit Care 2005;10(5):242–6.
[70] Pronovost PJ, Angus DC, Dorman T, et al. Physician staffing patterns and clinical outcomes in critically ill patients: a systematic review. JAMA 2002;288(17):2151–62.
[71] Kane SL, Weber RJ, Dasta JF. The impact of critical care pharmacists on enhancing patient outcomes. Intensive Care Med 2003;29(5):691–8.
[72] Leape LL, Cullen DJ, Clapp MD, et al. Pharmacist participation on physician rounds and adverse drug events in the intensive care unit. JAMA 1999;282(3):267–70 [erratum appears in JAMA 2000;283(10):1293].

[73] Raju TN, Kecskes S, Thornton JP, et al. Medication errors in neonatal and paediatric intensive-care units. Lancet 1989;2(8659):374–6.
[74] Flaatten H, Hevroy O. Errors in the intensive care unit (ICU). Experiences with an anonymous registration. Acta Anaesthesiol Scand 1999;43(6):614–7.
[75] Suresh G, Horbar JD, Plsek P, et al. Voluntary anonymous reporting of medical errors for neonatal intensive care. Pediatrics 2004;113(6):1609–18.
[76] Lesar TS, Briceland LL, Delcoure K, et al. Medication prescribing errors in a teaching hospital. JAMA 1990;263(17):2329–34.
[77] Folli HL, Poole RL, Benitz WE, et al. Medication error prevention by clinical pharmacists in two children's hospitals. Pediatrics 1987;79(5):718–22.
[78] Osmon S, Harris CB, Dunagan WC, et al. Reporting of medical errors: an intensive care unit experience. Crit Care Med 2004;32(3):727–33.
[79] Tisdale JE. Justifying a pediatric critical-care satellite pharmacy by medication-error reporting. Am J Hosp Pharm 1986;43(2):368–71.
[80] Schneider MP, Cotting J, Pannatier A. Evaluation of nurses' errors associated in the preparation and administration of medication in a pediatric intensive care unit. Pharm World Sci 1998;20(4):178–82.
[81] Donchin Y, Gopher D, Olin M, et al. A look into the nature and causes of human errors in the intensive care unit. Crit Care Med 1995;23(2):294–300.
[82] Dean BS, Barber ND. A validated, reliable method of scoring the severity of medication errors. Am J Health Syst Pharm 1999;56(1):57–62.
[83] Hartwig SC, Denger SD, Schneider PJ. Severity-indexed, incident report-based medication error-reporting program. Am J Hosp Pharm 1991;48(12):2611–6.

ELSEVIER
SAUNDERS

Crit Care Clin 22 (2006) 291–311

CRITICAL
CARE
CLINICS

Antimicrobial Resistance: Factors and Outcomes

Douglas N. Fish, PharmD[a,b,*], Martin J. Ohlinger, PharmD[c,d]

[a]*Department of Clinical Pharmacy, School of Pharmacy, University of Colorado Health Sciences Center, Campus Box C-238, 4200 East Ninth Avenue, Denver, CO 80262, USA*
[b]*Critical Care/Infectious Diseases, Department of Pharmacy, University of Colorado Hospital, Denver, CO 80262, USA*
[c]*Department of Pharmacy Practice, University of Toledo College of Pharmacy, Wolfe Hall, Suite 1246, Mail Stop 609 2801, West Bancroft Street, Toledo, OH 43606, USA*
[d]*Medical University of Ohio University Medical Center, Toledo, OH 43606, USA*

Patients often are admitted to the ICU for treatment of community-acquired or hospital-acquired infections, and many other patients require treatment for nosocomial infections acquired during their ICU stay. Because ICU patients experience high rates of infectious complications and are exposed to high rates of antimicrobial use [1,2], the emergence of antimicrobial resistance has made the appropriate use of antimicrobials a considerable challenge to clinicians. The difficulty in the use of antimicrobials lies in the need to balance two conflicting goals: (1) the provision of aggressive and appropriate antimicrobial therapy to treat infections adequately and (2) the avoidance of excessive antimicrobial use to limit the emergence and spread of antimicrobial resistance. This article briefly describes the scope of the resistance problem in critically ill patients, summarizes risk factors and outcomes associated with this resistance, and discusses strategies related to antibiotic use that potentially may limit or reduce resistance.

* Corresponding author. Department of Clinical Pharmacy, School of Pharmacy, University of Colorado Health Sciences Center, Campus Box C-238, 4200 East Ninth Avenue, Denver, CO 80262.
E-mail address: doug.fish@uchsc.edu (D.N. Fish).

0749-0704/06/$ – see front matter
doi:10.1016/j.ccc.2006.02.006

Antimicrobial resistance in intensive care units

It has been estimated that 50% to 60% of all nosocomial infections in the United States are caused by antibiotic-resistant bacteria [2]. Table 1 summarizes the overall prevalence and important trends in increasing resistance in the United States among selected pathogens and drug classes [1,3,4]. Much of the changing epidemiology of infection in the ICU has centered around the emergence of multidrug-resistant gram-positive organisms, such as methicillin-resistant *Staphylococcus aureus* (MRSA), vancomycin-resistant enterococci, and multidrug-resistant *Streptococcus pneumoniae,* as predominant pathogens in critically ill patients [1,3,5]. Although MRSA traditionally has been regarded as a hospital-acquired pathogen, this pathogen also has emerged as a common cause of community-acquired infections, with approximately 30% of all MRSA isolates now community-acquired in origin [6–8]. The increase in methicillin-resistant staphylococci has led to a heavy reliance on vancomycin and perhaps is related to the dramatic increase in vancomycin-resistant enterococci among ICU patients.

Antimicrobial resistance also continues to be an increasingly important problem among gram-negative bacilli. Of particular concern is the rapid spread of resistance mediated by extended-spectrum β-lactamases among organisms such as *Klebsiella pneumoniae* and *Escherichia coli*. Organisms that produce extended-spectrum β-lactamases are usually resistant to multiple antimicrobials, including third-generation (eg, ceftriaxone, ceftazidime) and fourth-generation (eg, cefepime) cephalosporins and aztreonam, [9,10] and are associated with high rates of resistance to aminoglycosides and fluoroquinolones [10,11]. Resistance of *Pseudomonas aeruginosa* to fluoroquinolones and imipenem also has increased rap-

Table 1
Antimicrobial resistance among selected nosocomial pathogens from ICU patients in the United States, 1998–2002 and 2003

Pathogen	Resistance rate, 1998–2002	Resistance rate, 2003	Percent change, 1998–2002 to 2003
Vancomycin-resistant enterococci	25.4	28.5	12
Methicillin-resistant *S aureus*	53.6	59.5	11
Methicillin-resistant coagulase-negative staphylococci	88.2	89.1	1
3GC-resistant *E coli**	5.8	5.8	0
3GC-resistant *K pneumoniae**	14	20.6	47
Imipenem-resistant *P aeruginosa*	18.3	21.1	15
Fluoroquinolone-resistant *P aeruginosa*	27	29.5	9
3GC-resistant *P aeruginosa*	26.6	31.9	20
3GC-resistant *Enterobacter* species	33	31.1	−6

Abbreviation: 3GC, third-generation cephalosporin (cefotaxime, ceftriaxone, or ceftazidime).

* Rates reflect nonsusceptibility (resistant and intermediate susceptibility).

Adapted from US Department of Public Health and Human Services, Public Health Service. National Nosocomial Infections Surveillance (NNIS) system report, data summary from January 1992 through June 2004, issued October 2004. Am J Infect Control 2004;32:470–85.

idly; nearly 10% of *P aeruginosa* isolates are now resistant to multiple drug classes, including cephalosporins, carbapenems, aminoglycosides, and fluoroquinolones [12]. Multidrug resistance also is common (approximately 25% of isolates) among strains of *Acinetobacter baumanii*. Fluoroquinolone resistance also is being increasingly reported among organisms such as *E coli* that are usually considered to be extremely susceptible to this class of drugs [4,13].

Although resistance to antifungal agents among *Candida* species usually is considered to be quite infrequent, a multicenter study of 50 hospitals in the United States found that 10% of *C albicans* isolates from bloodstream infections were resistant to fluconazole [14]. The relative frequency of fungal infections with *Candida krusei* and other strains with decreased susceptibility to azole antifungals also is increasing among critically ill patients [15].

Numerous factors are associated with high rates of antimicrobial resistance in the ICU. Chief among these is the heavy use of antimicrobials in critically ill patients. Many studies have identified an association between antimicrobial use and the subsequent development of resistance [16–21]. Use of antibiotics is associated with the emergence of resistance during therapy, but previous exposure also is a well-established risk factor for antimicrobial resistance [1,2, 16,22]. Increased resistance is related to several variables associated with the higher severity of illness found among ICU patients, including the presence of invasive devices, such as endotracheal tubes and intravascular and urinary catheters [2,23]; prolonged length of hospital stay [18,24,25]; immunosuppression [1]; malnutrition [1,2]; and ease of cross-transmission of antimicrobial-resistant pathogens owing to poor adherence of hospital personnel to infection control techniques, contamination of equipment, and frequent overcrowding of patients [1,26,27]. The increasing prevalence of antimicrobial-resistant pathogens among residents in long-term care facilities also is an important source for resistant bacteria in ICUs [1,2,5,22,28]. All of these various factors combine to make ICUs the epicenter of antimicrobial resistance in hospitalized patients [29].

Impact of resistance in critically ill patients

Infections caused by antimicrobial-resistant bacteria have been associated with higher mortality rates and longer length of ICU and hospital stays [30–33]. Increased mortality associated with infections caused by resistant bacteria may be explained partly by the increased likelihood that patients will receive inadequate antimicrobial treatment. Inadequate antimicrobial therapy, defined as the use of drugs with poor in vitro activity against the pathogen, has been shown in numerous studies to be significantly associated with increased mortality, increased hospital and ICU lengths of stay, increased duration of mechanical ventilation, and increased treatment costs [34–43]. Treatment with inadequate antimicrobial therapy is particularly problematic during the initial empiric treatment of infections when specific pathogens and antibiotic susceptibility information is not yet available [34,36,38–40].

In a study of 135 consecutive episodes of ventilator-associated pneumonia (VAP), no combination of even three antibiotics could be found that would provide adequate therapy in more than 88% of episodes [37]. It is logical to assume that selection of adequate empiric therapy becomes more difficult as the organisms become more resistant to antimicrobial therapy, and it has been shown in clinical studies that most inadequate treatment of nosocomial infections in the ICU is related to the presence of pathogens that are resistant to the selected antibiotics [34,37]. In the study of VAP, one quarter of all cases of inappropriate antimicrobial therapy in the ICU were caused by resistant gram-negative bacilli, and patients who received inappropriate therapy had significantly higher morbidity and mortality compared with patients treated appropriately (52% versus 12%) [37]. It has been shown in patients with nosocomial pneumonia that changing to more appropriate antibiotics when culture and susceptibility results became available (typically 48–72 hours after initiating therapy) did not lower mortality rates significantly compared with patients who received inadequate antibiotics for the entire duration of therapy [35]. The importance of antimicrobial resistance in terms of antimicrobial selection and patient outcomes cannot be overstated.

Basic principles of appropriate antimicrobial use

Although many of the issues regarding antimicrobial use in critically ill patients currently are centered on issues specifically related to antimicrobial resistance, adherence to basic principles of appropriate drug use is still crucial in overall optimization of drug therapy. These basic principles are summarized in Box 1 and include appropriate diagnostic considerations, selection of antimicrobials for empiric therapy, and selection of definitive antimicrobials (ie, based on culture and susceptibility information) for proven infections.

Diagnostic issues

A full discussion of issues related to the diagnosis of infection in ICU patients is beyond the scope of this article. These issues are nevertheless crucial in appropriately selecting antimicrobials for patients who require them and avoiding unnecessary or excessively prolonged use [44,45].

Selection of empiric drug therapy

As previously discussed, selection of inadequate therapy has been shown in numerous clinical studies to be associated with increased patient morbidity and mortality, and the risk of inadequate therapy often is related directly to rates of

Box 1. Basic principles of appropriate antimicrobial use in critically ill patients

Establish definitive diagnosis before initiating antimicrobials

1. Perform comprehensive clinical evaluation
2. Determine known or suspected site of infection
3. Perform appropriate diagnostic tests
4. Obtain appropriate specimens for culture and susceptibility testing
   - Gram stain of appropriate specimens
   - Evaluate cultures and Gram stains for colonization versus infection
5. Evaluate patient for noninfectious sources of fever
   - Hemorrhage
   - Inflammatory conditions
   - Medications
   - Metabolic conditions
   - Neoplasms
   - Thromboembolism

Initiate appropriate empiric antimicrobial therapy

1. Consider known/probable site of infection and most likely pathogens
2. Consider results of any previous diagnostic tests
   - Consider colonization versus infection when evaluating culture results
3. Consider rates of antimicrobial resistance among potential pathogens
   - Consider resistance among community-acquired and nosocomial pathogens
   - Consider differences in resistance patterns in ICU and among various units
4. Consider prior antimicrobial exposure and potential for selection of resistant pathogens
5. Consider need for combination antimicrobial therapy versus monotherapy
6. Initial therapy should be broad-spectrum, parenteral, and at appropriately aggressive doses
   - Consider pharmacokinetic properties of potentially used agents and potential alterations
   - Consider pharmacodynamic properties of potentially used agents

Consider age, organ dysfunction, and site of infection when determining proper dose
Consider potential drug-related adverse effects and toxicities
Consider potentially relevant drug-drug or drug–disease state interactions
Consider use of less expensive agents when appropriate

Change to appropriate definitive drug therapy when possible

1. Monitor culture and susceptibility test results
2. Spectrum of antimicrobial activity of selected agents should be as narrow as possible when pathogens is known
3. Consider need for combination antimicrobial therapy versus monotherapy
4. Therapy should be at appropriately aggressive doses
   Consider pharmacokinetic properties of potentially used agents and potential alterations
   Consider pharmacodynamic properties of potentially used agents
   Consider age, organ dysfunction, and site of infection when determining proper dose
   Consider potential drug-related adverse effects and toxicities
   Consider potentially relevant drug-drug or drug–disease state interactions
   Consider use of less expensive agents when appropriate

Consider use of oral antimicrobials when appropriate

1. Patients clinically responding to parenteral therapy
2. Patients have functional gastrointestinal tracts
3. Suitable oral alternatives to parenteral therapy available

Perform careful patient monitoring for duration of antimicrobial therapy

1. Evaluate for clinical resolution of signs and symptoms and evidence of response to therapy
2. Evaluate for changes in organ function that may require change in drug dosing regimen
3. Monitor serum drug concentrations when appropriate
4. Evaluate for drug-related adverse effects and toxicities
5. Evaluate for potential adverse drug interactions

Carefully reassess patients who seem to be failing antimicrobial therapy

1. Evaluate patient for unidentified or new sources or sites of infection or superinfection
2. Obtain additional specimens for culture and susceptibility testing
3. Evaluate drug regimen for proper spectrum of activity against known or presumed pathogens
   Consider emergence of antibiotic resistance among certain pathogens (e.g., *P aeruginosa*)
4. Evaluate drug regimen for proper dosing of individual antimicrobial agents
   Consider pharmacokinetic and pharmacodynamic properties of agents and potential need for increased daily doses or alternative dosing methods

Limit duration of therapy when possible

1. Short courses are desired over long courses in patients who have responded promptly to antimicrobial therapy
2. In patients with no documented infection or pathogens, discontinue antimicrobials after appropriate course of therapy and assess continued need for treatment

antimicrobial resistance in certain pathogens [34–40]. As shown in Box 1, numerous factors are important to consider when choosing drugs for initial empiric therapy and the manner in which these drugs will be used. In general, empiric antimicrobial regimens for critically ill patients should be sufficiently broad-spectrum in pharmacologic activity to cover the most likely pathogens, initiated promptly, and given in relatively high doses when the presence of any significant renal or hepatic dysfunction is accounted for.

Because resistance rates for even the same organism (eg, *E coli*) may be different when isolated from community-acquired versus nosocomial sources, clinicians should be familiar with resistance patterns of key pathogens involved in community-acquired and nosocomial infections to choose appropriate antibiotics. Although antibiograms summarizing drug susceptibilities of key pathogens are available in most institutions, they often do not differentiate between ICU and non-ICU isolates. Resistance rates are often much higher among ICU isolates because of heavier antimicrobial use and the presence of more risk factors for resistance [46–48]. Clinicians should be aware of differences in susceptibilities between different ICUs (eg, medical, surgical, trauma) when such information is available.

Selection of definitive drug therapy

Clinicians must use results of culture and susceptibility tests when available to reassess and make appropriate changes to empiric drug regimens. Antimicrobial regimens should be selected that provide suitable activity against identified pathogens, while using the fewest required number of drugs and narrowing the spectrum of antimicrobial activity as much as possible. It is common for patients to be treated empirically for the entire duration of therapy because of the frequent inability to identify the site of infection, negative culture results, cultures suspected to be positive for colonizing organisms rather than pathogens, or other reasons. Rational antimicrobial therapy dictates, however, that culture and susceptibility information must be used in the selection of more definitive antimicrobial therapy when such information is available and believed to be reliable. It is inappropriate to continue empirically selected drug regimens simply because the patient is clinically responding to present therapy and the clinician is unwilling to make a change of any kind. This practice often results in excessively broad therapy being used for long durations, both of which are significant risk factors for resistance.

Strategies to reduce antimicrobial resistance

Various strategies have been used to decrease resistance through improved antimicrobial use, including the appropriate application of pharmacokinetic and pharmacodynamic principles to antimicrobial use, aggressive dosing of antimicrobials, use of broad-spectrum or combination antimicrobial therapy, decreased duration of therapy, hospital formulary–based or targeted antimicrobial restrictions, use of antimicrobial protocols and guidelines, scheduled antimicrobial rotation or "cycling," and antimicrobial management programs. These strategies and the evidence for or against their routine use are discussed in detail in the remainder of this article.

Application of pharmacokinetic and pharmacodynamic principles

Ineffective antimicrobial dosing is a common yet often unrecognized factor associated with clinical treatment failures and an increased probability of the emergence of resistance. Antimicrobials are selected based primarily on their pharmacologic activity against presumed or documented pathogens. Because of the severity and high risk of morbidity and mortality associated with infections in critically ill patients, however, optimization of antimicrobial therapy requires that drugs also be dosed in a manner that maximizes their pharmacologic activity, while minimizing the risk of adverse effects and toxicities.

The application of pharmacodynamic principles combines information regarding the pharmacologic activity of an antibiotic (based on minimum inhibitory concentrations [MIC] of a drug for a target pathogen) with information regarding the drug's pharmacokinetic properties. Pharmacodynamic considerations combine MIC-defined activity and pharmacokinetic properties to make predictions regarding the drug's probable efficacy in the treatment of infections, and appropriate pharmacodynamic considerations allow clinical variables, such as drug dosing regimens, to be manipulated to increase this probability of clinical cure [49]. Drugs such as β-lactams, aztreonam, carbapenems, and vancomycin are characterized as concentration-independent antibiotics, also known as time-dependent drugs, and their efficacy is based on maintaining concentrations of the agent above the MIC of the organism for prolonged periods [49]. Use of continuous antibiotic infusions has been promoted for time-dependent drugs to optimize their pharmacodynamic properties and minimize the risk of bacterial resistance [49,50]. Numerous in vitro investigations and clinical trials evaluating continuous infusion of penicillin, ceftazidime, cefepime, piperacillin, imipenem, meropenem, and vancomycin have been published [51–55]. Concentration-dependent antibiotics, particularly aminoglycosides and fluoroquinolones, exert their maximal antibacterial activities when peak drug concentrations are well above the MIC of the organism [49]. Newer dosing strategies also have been employed for concentration-dependent antimicrobials to optimize their pharmacodynamic properties and maximize efficacy. Such strategies include the use of extended-interval dosing regimens for aminoglycosides and the use of high doses of fluoroquinolones to achieve high concentrations relative to the pathogen MICs [56–58].

Studies have shown that dosing strategies that optimize pharmacodynamic properties of antibiotics often result in improved bacterial eradication, decreased mortality, and decreased length of ICU and hospital stays. The ability of these pharmacodynamically based dosing regimens to prevent or delay the development of resistance in the clinical setting is still uncertain, however. Most published trials have been structured to measure short-term efficacy outcomes, such as those mentioned here, but have not addressed the emergence of resistance in patients during treatment or effects on institutional resistance patterns over longer periods. Few studies regarding optimization of antimicrobial pharmacodynamics in the clinical setting measured resistance, and no difference in rates of resistance between the treatment groups was reported [59].

The application of pharmacodynamic principles to the ICU patient is complicated by the potential for significantly altered drug pharmacokinetics in the critically ill patient [60]. Larger volumes of distribution secondary to volume overload, decreased serum protein concentrations leading to decreased protein binding, decreased metabolism and clearance owing to organ dysfunction or hypoperfusion, and increased metabolism and clearance owing to hypermetabolic states all have been described in ICU patients, and all may lead to clinically significant changes in antimicrobial pharmacokinetics [60]. Despite the inherent challenges in critically ill patients, optimization of antibiotic dosing based on better characterization of pharmacokinetic alterations in ICU patients and appropriate application of pharmacodynamic principles offers significant potential for improving patient outcomes, while reducing the problem of antimicrobial resistance.

Aggressive dosing of antimicrobials

Because of the severity of infections in critically ill patients and the variability in pharmacokinetics and tissue penetration, the general recommendation for dosing of antimicrobials in ICU patients is to use aggressive dosing strategies. Low doses of antibiotics may fail to eradicate pathogens and predispose to the development of resistance. Conversely, the use of high doses potentially compensates for pharmacokinetic alterations that may be present, increases the likelihood that patients are receiving adequate drug to achieve pharmacodynamic goals of antimicrobial use, and may be associated with higher probabilities of clinical success and decreased resistance. Use of high doses also may put patients at higher risk of drug-related adverse events, however, partially as a result of the pharmacokinetic variability in drug distribution and elimination. Although drug dosing should be aggressive, it also must be based on appropriate clinical considerations involving relevant issues, such as drug toxicities, presence of renal or hepatic dysfunction that may lead to drug accumulation, the presumed site of infection and the ability of the drug to achieve adequate concentrations in that site, susceptibilities of presumed or documented pathogens, and pharmacodynamic properties of the drugs in question.

Broad-spectrum versus narrow-spectrum therapy and monotherapy versus combination therapy

Empiric therapy for most nosocomial infections in critically ill patients should be broad and provide gram-positive and gram-negative activity. Antimicrobial combinations that are active against a variety of potential pathogens may help reduce the likelihood of inappropriate therapy owing to bacterial resistance. The need for appropriate initial therapy must be carefully balanced, however, against the risk of increased resistance as a consequence of unnecessary drug exposure. Empiric therapy should be adjusted promptly based on clinical response of the patient and culture and sensitivity reports. Even when initial reports show an isolate is susceptible to the prescribed therapy, clinical failure dictates a change in antimicrobial therapy because resistance may be inducible, and the expression of such treatment-emergent resistance may not be observed until after therapy has been initiated. In patients who respond to initial therapy, de-escalation (narrowing of spectrum or reduction in number of antimicrobials) of therapy is desirable. De-escalation decreases antimicrobial pressure for the development of resistance and potentially may lower the incidence of adverse drug events and treatment cost [61,62].

Data supporting the use of combination antibiotic therapy for initial empiric therapy or definitive treatment for nosocomial infections are inconsistent [63,64]. Many studies have compared monotherapy with combination therapy for the management of nosocomial pneumonia, VAP, or bacteremia [65–73].

Multidrug resistance may occur in early-onset (ie, <7 days of mechanical ventilation) or late-onset pneumonia [74]. Resistance is almost exclusively associated, however, with either longer durations of hospital or ICU stay (or residence in a health care institutional facility) or prior antibiotic therapy. Patients not at risk for multidrug resistance who develop early-onset nosocomial pneumonia or VAP may be treated adequately with monotherapy without great risk of treatment failure secondary to resistance. Much of the evidence from trials of monotherapy versus combination therapy of VAP fails to document benefits of combination therapy. Many of these trials were performed, however, before the emergence of the current problems of frequent multidrug resistance. Although severe infections caused by multidrug-resistant *P aeruginosa, Klebsiella,* or *Acinetobacter* often are treated with combination therapy, conclusive clinical data supporting this as routine practice are lacking. In vitro studies show synergistic activity for combinations of an antipseudomonal β-lactam plus an aminoglycoside or fluoroquinolone against *P aeruginosa* and other nonfermenting gram-negative organisms [75,76]. In vivo data clearly supporting the role of synergy and routine use of combination therapy are mostly lacking, however.

A retrospective review of 115 patients treated with monotherapy or combination therapy for *P aeruginosa* bacteremia evaluated early mortality (before receipt of the culture and sensitivity data) and late mortality (after receipt of the culture and sensitivity data to day 30) [39]. Using multivariate analysis, late mortality was significantly higher in patients who received adequate empiric monotherapy or inadequate therapy compared with patients who received adequate empiric combination therapy. The clinical importance of resistance was discussed in the article, but the contributions of resistance to outcomes observed in the study were not specifically analyzed. Nonetheless, one may hypothesize that combination therapy seems to have conferred a benefit in that the use of more than one agent may have resulted in a higher likelihood of patients receiving at least one agent with activity against the pathogen. Such a conclusion also may be supported by the finding that patients in the study who received adequate definitive combination therapy did not have a better outcome than the patients who received adequate definitive monotherapy. Although this was a retrospective review, it is one of the few studies to show a mortality benefit associated with combination therapy for *P aeruginosa* infections.

Resistance in complicated intra-abdominal infections also is problematic because many of these infections are polymicrobial and may involve more difficult nosocomial pathogens. Montravers and colleagues [77] showed a high prevalence of resistant microbial flora after intra-abdominal surgery with associated increases in treatment failure and mortality. Complicated intra-abdominal infections may require the use of combination antimicrobial therapy.

Duration of therapy

The optimal duration of therapy for many infectious diseases, particularly in ICU patients, is poorly defined. The duration of antimicrobial therapy often is based on limited or old data, extrapolated from different patient populations or disease states, or based entirely on expert opinion. More recent investigations have evaluated whether shortening the duration of antimicrobial therapy decreases the emergence of resistance, while maintaining clinical efficacy, and at least two studies in nosocomial pneumonia have challenged the notion of the requirement for long durations of therapy. Singh and colleagues [78] randomized ICU patients with an equivocal diagnosis of VAP based on the clinical pulmonary infection score to ciprofloxacin, 400 mg intravenously every 8 hours for 3 days, or therapy left to the discretion of the attending physician (ie, control group). The clinical pulmonary infection score was determined again at the end of 3 days of ciprofloxacin therapy, and antibiotics were discontinued in patients with a continued equivocal diagnosis of pneumonia (ie, short-course treatment) or continued in patients with a clear diagnosis of VAP. Patients in the short-course and control groups had similar clinical pulmonary infection scores, but the short-course treatment group received 6.8 fewer days of antibiotics ($P = .0001$), costing 60% less than controls; stayed in the ICU 5.3 fewer days ($P = .04$); had a 13% lower absolute mortality rate (18% versus 31%; $P = .06$); and had a 24% absolute reduction in rates of superinfection and antibiotic resistance (14% versus 38% for controls; $P = .017$) [78].

A multicenter study comparing 8 days with 15 days of antimicrobial therapy for VAP showed that patients treated for the shorter duration had similar rates of mortality, infection recurrence, and ventilator-free days and decreased number of organ failure–free days and length of ICU stay compared with patients receiving the longer course of therapy [79]. Only patients with VAP caused by nonfermenting gram-negative bacilli, including *P aeruginosa,* had higher infection recurrence rates after 8 days of therapy compared with 15-day therapy. In patients experiencing recurrent infections, the emergence of multidrug resistance was significantly less common in patients who received the 8-day regimen compared with patients who received 15 days of therapy.

More recently, the success of an antibiotic discontinuation policy for clinically suspected VAP was reported [80]. Patients were assigned to have the duration of antibiotic treatment for VAP determined by an antibiotic discontinuation policy (discontinuation group) or their treating physician teams (conventional group). Although the severity of illness and likelihood of VAP were similar between the groups, the duration of antibiotic treatment was statistically shorter among patients in the discontinuation group compared with patients in the conventional management group (6 days versus 8 days; $P = .001$). Occurrence of secondary episodes of VAP, ICU length of stay, and hospital mortality were similar between the two groups. Changes in antibiotic resistance rates were not assessed.

Antibiotic formularies

Formulary-driven restriction of drugs or drug classes is a common method of controlling antimicrobial use within an institution. Formulary-based restrictions historically have been used to control drug costs; they also may reduce rates of adverse effects of high-risk agents [81]. More recently, antimicrobial restrictions have been used in an attempt to decrease overall emergence of antimicrobial resistance within an institution or to control acute outbreaks of resistance affecting specific drugs and pathogens [17,82–84]. The effectiveness of antimicrobial formulary restrictions in reducing overall levels of resistance has not been shown consistently. It has been argued that formulary restrictions alone can cause intense selective pressure from a smaller number of agents and may promote the emergence of resistance, rather than prevent it [81]. Antibiotic restrictions that are instituted in response to specific outbreaks of antibiotic-resistant infections, together with appropriate infection control measures, have been shown to manage specific resistance problems successfully [82–84]. It also has been shown, however, that restriction of a drug in response to a resistance issue may cause other resistance problems affecting other drugs [17]. This phenomenon is sometimes referred to as "squeezing the balloon" because the enforcement of antimicrobial restrictions leads to new selective pressures, which may solve the original problem effectively, but cause the development of new resistance [85]. A classic example involved restriction of ceftazidime and increased use of imipenem in response to an outbreak of ceftazidime-resistant *K pneumoniae*; although ceftazidime resistance among *K pneumoniae* isolates was decreased effectively by 44%, the rates of imipenem-resistant *P aeruginosa* significantly increased by 69% [17]. Although antimicrobial restrictions may be effective in reducing drug costs and limiting specific outbreaks of resistant infections, the emphasis must be on appropriate and rational drug use, rather than relying on such restrictions to overcome resistance problems.

Guidelines and protocols for antimicrobial use

The use of guidelines, practice parameters, clinical pathways, or protocols is associated with more appropriate medication use, improved patient outcomes, fewer adverse events and errors, and better resource use for many disease states, including infectious diseases. The Infectious Diseases Society of America and the American Thoracic Society published joint consensus guidelines for the management of nosocomial pneumonia, VAP, and health care–associated pneumonia [86]. Much of this document is focused on treatment issues related to emerging multidrug-resistant pathogens, including *P aeruginosa, Klebsiella, Enterobacter, Serratia, Acinetobacter, Stenotrophomonas maltophilia, Burkholderia cepacia,* MRSA, *and S pneumoniae*. A previous consensus paper from an international expert panel was published in 2001 [87]. Regarding resistance, this panel of experts from Europe and Latin America stated, "All the peers agreed that the pathogens causing VAP and multiresistance patterns in their ICUs were substantially different than those . . . in the United States," reinforcing the need to use local susceptibility data in the development of guidelines or protocols for general use in institutions and the selection of appropriate antibiotic therapy for individual patients.

Ibrahim and colleagues [88] investigated the effect of a clinical protocol for the management of VAP. The trial prospectively followed 50 patients before implementation of the protocol (control group) and 52 patients after protocol implementation, focusing primarily on the appropriateness of antimicrobial therapy and reducing unnecessary antimicrobial use in this patient population. Compared with the control group, the protocol-driven group received adequate empiric therapy more often (94% versus 48%), received significantly fewer days of antimicrobial therapy (8.6 days versus 14.8 days), and had a lower incidence of recurrent VAP (8% versus 24%). The authors did not report a difference in hospital length of stay, ICU length of stay, or mortality between the two groups. Regarding resistance, although no differences in susceptibility patterns were found during the trial, the most common reason for inadequate antimicrobial treatment during both phases of the study continued to be the isolation of resistant pathogens, such as MRSA, *P aeruginosa*, *Serratia marcescens, S maltophilia,* and *Acinetobacter*.

Programs for restriction of target antibiotics and antibiotic cycling

Institution-wide programs for improving antimicrobial use and decreasing resistance may be as simple as enforcing formulary restrictions or as complex as implementing scheduled antibiotic rotations. Resistance is one of the most common reasons cited for restriction of an antimicrobial or class of antimicrobial agents. Targeted antimicrobials may be restricted based on differences in efficacy, usage criteria, resistance patterns, cost, or other factors. Such criteria may be used to prioritize usage within a class of antimicrobial agents or across different classes. The scheduled rotation of antibiotic usage within institutions also has been studied for several years [89–93]. Early studies focused mainly on detecting changes in resistance patterns associated with rotation programs. Later studies also evaluated associations between antibiotic rotation and patient outcomes, including mortality. The rationale for antibiotic rotation (or cycling) in institutions as a whole or specifically within the ICU is to limit bacterial exposure to certain antimicrobials over a defined period, decreasing the emergence of resistance or delaying the time required for organisms to become resistant to those drugs.

Researchers at a large medical center with significant *P aeruginosa* resistance to β-lactams implemented a pharmacist-facilitated, institution-wide antimicrobial restriction program [94]. All orders for restricted antimicrobials (eg, antipseudomonal β-lactams, amikacin, tobramycin, fluoroquinolones) were prospectively reviewed for appropriateness, and therapy was continued or modified accordingly. The results of this study are particularly noteworthy in that a change in the usage of a single agent (ceftazidime) was associated with significant changes in the *P aeruginosa* susceptibilities of multiple agents, even beyond the restricted agent's antimicrobial class. The use of ceftazidime declined by 44% during the first 4 years of the restriction program, carbapenem use declined slightly, piperacillin use did not change significantly, and aztreonam use increased by 57%. Although *P aeruginosa* resistance to ceftazidime decreased from 24% to 12%, similar declines in *P aeruginosa* resistance were observed for imipenem (20–12%), piperacillin (32–18%), and even aztreonam (30–16%) [95]. These findings may seem contrary to the "squeezing the balloon" effect previously discussed. Although the initial resistance problem identified was primarily that of a single pathogen and agent (*P aeruginosa* and ceftazidime), however, the restriction program encouraged appropriate use of a broad variety of antimicrobials and did not focus exclusively on limiting the use of one agent.

Raymond and colleagues [91] evaluated an antibiotic rotation program in a surgical ICU among patients with pneumonia, peritonitis, or sepsis. The 1-year period of antibiotic rotation was compared with the previous 1-year period in which antibiotic use was at the discretion of the attending physician. Fluoroquinolones, cephalosporins, carbapenems, and β-lactam/β-lactamase inhibitor combinations were involved in the rotation. Antibiotic rotation occurred quarterly, and use of specific agents varied with the type of infection. Attributable mortality decreased significantly during the protocol-driven period, from 56% to 35%; rates of resistant gram-positive infections decreased from 14.6 to 7.8 infections per 100 ICU admissions; and rates of gram-negative infections decreased from 7.7 to 2.5 infections per 100 ICU admissions. Finally, stepwise logistic regression analysis of factors associated with mortality identified antibiotic rotation as an independent predictor of survival.

Another study evaluated rates of VAP caused by gram-negative bacilli in a medical ICU throughout a 7-year period [92]. During the first 2 years, no protocol for antimicrobial use for VAP was used. For the next 5 years, a 1-month antibiotic rotation schedule was implemented. The incidence of VAP was significantly lower during the 5 years of the antibiotic rotation program compared with the initial 2-year period. Although the incidence of infection with organisms considered potentially multidrug resistant (eg, *P aeruginosa, B cepacia, Acinetobacter*) increased, antibiotic susceptibilities nevertheless improved. Gram-negative resistance rates remained unchanged overall.

Although these and other studies showed promising results [89,90,93], they have not been altogether consistent in the demonstrated benefits of antibiotic cycling programs, and many important questions regarding antibiotic cycling have not been addressed adequately. These questions concern which antibiotics or classes are most appropriate to cycle, whether the specific order of agents in the cycle is important, the optimal scheduled time between changes in cycled antibiotics, and the long-term effectiveness of antibiotic cycling. Additional research is needed to answer these and other relevant questions, although the concept itself seems promising as a means of reducing resistance.

Antimicrobial management programs

Hospital-based antimicrobial management programs (or "antimicrobial stewardship programs") consist of an organized approach of combining educational efforts with various restriction programs [95]. Antimicrobial management programs aim to improve the overall treatment of infectious diseases and antimicrobial use within the institution by coordinating and integrating efforts to detect and monitor rates of specific infections and the prevalence of resistance among key pathogens, and also to improve the appropriateness of antimicrobial use by instituting and enforcing various restriction programs [95,96]. Because of their nature, antimicrobial management programs often are directed by multidisciplinary teams consisting of infectious disease physicians, clinical pharmacists, infection control nurses or physicians, microbiologists, and other interested parties. The education of antibiotic prescribers within the institution is usually a key component. Incorporation of formulary and target drug restriction programs, antibiotic preapproval programs, and development of drug use policies and guidelines all are elements that also may be useful in specific institutions. Although the long-term impact of such antimicrobial management programs on reducing endemic resistance within an institution has not yet been well documented, such programs have been documented to be effective in dealing with outbreaks of multidrug-resistant pathogens, and it is presumed these programs are effective in improving endemic resistance as well [95,96].

Summary

Antimicrobial resistance within the ICU continues to be an ever-increasing problem, characterized by increasing overall resistance rates among gram-negative and gram-positive pathogens and increased frequency of multidrug-resistant organisms. Basic principles of appropriate drug selection for empiric and definitive therapy are still valid and must be emphasized in an effort to improve patient outcomes, while reducing resistance. Many other specific strategies have been recommended to decrease problems of resistance through improved use of antimicrobials, including appropriate application of pharmacokinetic and pharmacodynamic principles to guide antimicrobial use, aggressive dosing of antimicrobials, use of broad-spectrum and combination antimicrobial therapy, minimizing the duration of antimicrobial therapy, formulary-based antimicrobial restrictions, use of antimicrobial protocols and guidelines, programs for restriction of target antimicrobials, scheduled antimicrobial rotation or cycling, and use of antimicrobial management programs. Although the long-term effects of any one of these strategies likely would not be optimal to control resistance, combinations of various approaches offer the best potential for effectively intervening in and reducing the spread of resistant pathogens in critically ill patients.

References

[1] Fridkin SK, Gaynes RP. Antimicrobial resistance in intensive care units. Clin Chest Med 1999;20:303–16.
[2] Weinstein RA. Nosocomial infection update. Emerg Infect Dis 1998;4:416–20.
[3] US Department of Public Health and Human Services, Public Health Service. National Nosocomial Infections Surveillance (NNIS) system report, data summary from January 1992 through June 2004, issued October 2004. Am J Infect Control 2004;32:470–85.

[4] Neuhauser MM, Weinstein RA, Rydman R, et al. Antibiotic resistance among gram-negative bacilli in US intensive care units. Implications for fluoroquinolone use. JAMA 2003;289:885–8.
[5] Jones RN. Resistance patterns among nosocomial pathogens: trends over the past few years. Chest 2001;119(2 suppl):397S–404S.
[6] Bukharie H, Abdelhadi M, Saeed I, et al. Emergence of methicillin-resistant *Staphylococcus aureus* as a community pathogen. Diagn Microbiol Infect Dis 2001;40:1–4.
[7] Salgado CD, Farr BM, Calfee DP. Community-acquired methicillin-resistant *Staphylococcus aureus*: a meta-analysis of prevalence and risk factors. Clin Infect Dis 2003;36:131–9.
[8] Eady AE, Cove JH. Staphylococcal resistance revisited: community-acquired methicillin resistant *Staphylococcus aureus*—an emerging problem for the management of skin and soft tissue infections. Curr Opin Infect Dis 2003;16:103–24.
[9] Bush K. New β-lactamases in gram-negative bacteria: diversity and impact on the selection of antimicrobial therapy. Clin Infect Dis 2001;32:1085–9.
[10] Paterson DL, Ko W-C, Von Gottberg A, et al. Antibiotic therapy for *Klebsiella pneumoniae* bacteremia: implications of production of extended-spectrum β-lactamases. Clin Infect Dis 2003; 39:31–7.
[11] Paterson DL, Mulazimoglu L, Casellas JM, et al. Epidemiology of ciprofloxacin resistance and its relationship to extended-spectrum beta-lactamase production in *Klebsiella pneumoniae* isolates causing bacteremia. Clin Infect Dis 2000;30:473–8.
[12] Karlowsky JA, Draghi DC, Jones ME, et al. Surveillance for antimicrobial susceptibility among clinical isolates of *Pseudomonas aeruginosa* and *Acinetobacter baumanii* from hospitalized patients in the United States, 1998 to 2001. Antimicrob Agents Chemother 2003;47:1681–8.
[13] Zervos MJ, Hershberger E, Nicolau DP, et al. Relationship between fluoroquinolone use and changes in susceptibility to fluoroquinolones of selected pathogens in 10 United States teaching hospitals, 1991–2000. Clin Infect Dis 2003;37:1643–8.
[14] Pfaller MA, Jones RN, Messer SA, et al. National surveillance of nosocomial blood stream infection due to *Candida albicans*: frequency of occurrence and antifungal susceptibility in the SCOPE program. Diagn Microbiol Infect Dis 1998;31:327–32.
[15] Abi-Said D, Anaissie E, Uzon O, et al. The epidemiology of hematogenous candidiasis caused by different *Candida* species. Clin Infect Dis 1997;24:1122–8.
[16] Rello J, Ausina V, Ricart M, et al. Impact of previous antimicrobial therapy on the etiology and outcome of ventilator-associated pneumonia. Chest 1993;104:1230–5.
[17] Rahal JJ, Urban C, Horn D, et al. Class restriction of cephalosporin use to control total cephalosporin resistance in nosocomial *Klebsiella*. JAMA 1998;280:1233–7.
[18] Trouillet J-L, Chastre J, Vuagnat A, et al. Ventilator-associated pneumonia caused by potentially drug-resistant bacteria. Am J Respir Crit Care Med 1998;157:531–9.
[19] Marshall C, Wolfe R, Kossman T, et al. Risk factors for acquisition of methicillin-resistant *Staphylococcus aureus* (MRSA) by trauma patients in the intensive care unit. J Hosp Infect 2004;57:245–52.
[20] Paramythiotou E, Lucet J-C, Timsit J-F, et al. Acquisition of multidrug-resistant *Pseudomonas aeruginosa* in patients in intensive care units: role of antibiotics with antipseudomonal activity. Clin Infect Dis 2004;38:670–7.
[21] Lee S-O, Kim NJ, Choi S-H, et al. Risk factors for acquisition of imipenem-resistant *Acinetobacter baumanii*: a case-control study. Antimicrob Agents Chemother 2004;48:224–8.
[22] Kollef MH, Fraser VJ. Antibiotic resistance in the intensive care unit. Ann Intern Med 2001; 134:298–314.
[23] Jarvis WR, Edwards JR, Culver DH, et al. Nosocomial infection rates in adult and pediatric intensive care units in the United States. Am J Med 1991;91(suppl 3B):185S–91S.
[24] Albrich WC, Angstwurm M, Bader L, Gartner R. Drug resistance in intensive care units. Infection 1999;27(suppl 2):S19–23.
[25] Bonten MJ, Slaughter S, Hayden MK, et al. External sources of vancomycin-resistant enterococci for intensive care units. Crit Care Med 1998;26:2001–4.
[26] Fridkin SK, Pear SM, Williamson TH, et al. The role of understaffing in central venous catheter-associated bloodstream infections. Infect Control Hosp Epidemiol 1996;17:150–8.

[27] Alfieri N, Ramotar K, Armstrong P, et al. Two consecutive outbreaks of *Stenotrophomonas maltophilia* (*Xanthomonas maltophilia*) in an intensive-care unit defined by restriction fragment-length polymorphism typing. Infect Control Hosp Epidemiol 1999;20:553–6.
[28] Wiener J, Quinn JP, Bradford PA, et al. Multiple antibiotic-resistant *Klebsiella* and *Escherichia coli* in nursing homes. JAMA 1999;281:517–23.
[29] Archibald L, Phillips L, Monnet D, et al. Antimicrobial resistance in isolates from inpatients and outpatients in the United States: increasing importance of the intensive care unit. Clin Infect Dis 1997;24:211–5.
[30] Holemberg SD, Solomon SL, Blake PA. Health and economic impact of antimicrobial resistance. Rev Infect Dis 1987;9:1065–78.
[31] Ascar JF. Consequences of bacterial resistance to antibiotics in medical practice. Clin Infect Dis 1997;24(suppl):S17–8.
[32] Carmeli Y, Troillet N, Karchmer AW, Samore MH. Health and economic outcomes of antibiotic resistance in *Pseudomonas aeruginosa*. Arch Intern Med 1999;159:1127–32.
[33] Rello J, Torres A, Ricart M, et al. Ventilator-associated pneumonia by *Staphylococcus aureus*: comparison of methicillin-resistant and methicillin-sensitive episodes. Am J Respir Crit Care Med 1994;150(6 pt 1):1545–9.
[34] Alvarez-Lerma F, ICU-Acquired Pneumonia Study Group. Modification of empiric antibiotic treatment in patients with pneumonia acquired in the intensive care unit. Intensive Care Med 1996;22:387–94.
[35] Luna CM, Vujacich P, Niederman MS, et al. Impact of BAL data on the therapy and outcome of ventilator-associated pneumonia. Chest 1997;111:676–85.
[36] Leibovici L, Shraga I, Drucker M, et al. The benefit of appropriate empirical antibiotic treatment in patients with bloodstream infection. J Intern Med 1998;244:379–86.
[37] Kollef MH, Sherman G, Ward S, Fraser VJ. Inadequate antimicrobial treatment of infections: a risk factor for hospital mortality among critically ill patients. Chest 1999;115:462–74.
[38] Garnacho-Montero J, Garcia-Garmendia JL, Barrero-Almodovar A, et al. Impact of adequate empiric antibiotic therapy on the outcome of patients admitted to the intensive care unit with sepsis. Crit Care Med 2003;31:2742–51.
[39] Chamot E, Boffi El Amari E, Rohner P, Van Delden C. Effectiveness of combination antimicrobial therapy for *Pseudomonas aeruginosa* bacteremia. Antimicrob Agents Chemother 2003; 47:2756–64.
[40] MacArthur RD, Miller M, Albertson T, et al. Adequacy of early empiric antibiotic treatment and survival in severe sepsis: experience from the MONARCS trial. Clin Infect Dis 2004;38:284–8.
[41] Lautenbach E, Metlay JP, Bilker WB, et al. Association between fluoroquinolone resistance and mortality in *Escherichia coli* and *Klebsiella pneumoniae* infections: the role of inadequate empirical antimicrobial therapy. Clin Infect Dis 2005;41:923–9.
[42] Cosgrove SE, Youlin Q, Kaye KS, et al. The impact of methicillin resistance in *Staphylococcus aureus* bacteremia on patient outcomes: mortality, length of stay, and hospital charges. Infect Control Hosp Epidemiol 2005;26:166–74.
[43] Cosgrove SE. The relationship between antimicrobial resistance and patient outcomes: mortality, length of hospital stay, and health care costs. Clin Infect Dis 2006;42(suppl 2):S82–9.
[44] Kollef MH, Micek ST. Strategies to prevent antimicrobial resistance in the intensive care unit. Crit Care Med 2005;33:1845–53.
[45] Salgado CD, O'Grady N, Farr BM. Prevention and control of antimicrobial-resistant infections in intensive care patients. Crit Care Med 2005;33:2373–82.
[46] Pierson CL, Friedman BA. Comparison of susceptibility to beta-lactam antimicrobial agents among bacteria isolated from intensive care units. Diagn Microbiol Infect Dis 1992;15(suppl 2): 19S–30S.
[47] Campbell JR, Zaccaria E, Mason Jr EO, Baker LJ. Epidemiological analysis defining concurrent outbreaks of *Serratia marcescens* and methicillin-resistant *Staphylococcus aureus* in a neonatal intensive-care unit. Infect Control Hosp Epidemiol 1998;19:942–8.
[48] Husni RN, Goldstein LS, Arroliga AC, et al. Risk factors for an outbreak of multi-drug-resistant *Acinetobacter* nosocomial pneumonia among intubated patients. Chest 1999;115:1378–82.

[49] Craig WA. Pharmacokinetic/pharmacodynamic parameters: rationale for antibacterial dosing of mice and men. Clin Infect Dis 1998;26:1–12.
[50] Craig WA. Interrelationship between pharmacokinetics and pharmacodynamics in determining dosage regimens for broad-spectrum cephalosporins. Diagn Microbiol Infect Dis 1995;22: 89–96.
[51] Thalhammer F, Traunmuller F, El Menyawi I, et al. Continuous infusion versus intermittent administration of meropenem in critically ill patients. J Antimicrob Chemother 1999;43: 523–7.
[52] Hanes SD, Wood GC, Herring V, et al. Intermittent and continuous ceftazidime infusion for critically ill trauma patients. Am J Surg 2000;179:436–40.
[53] McNabb JJ, Nightingale CH, Quintiliani R, Nicolau DP. Cost-effectiveness of ceftazidime by continuous infusion versus intermittent infusion for nosocomial pneumonia. Pharmacotherapy 2001;21:549–55.
[54] Grant EM, Kuti JL, Nicolau DP, et al. Clinical efficacy and pharmacoeconomics of a continuous-infusion piperacillin-tazobactam program in a large community teaching hospital. Pharmacotherapy 2002;22:471–83.
[55] Boselli E, Breilh D, Duflo F, et al. Steady-state plasma and intrapulmonary concentrations of cefepime administered in continuous infusion in critically ill patients with severe nosocomial pneumonia. Crit Care Med 2003;31:2102–6.
[56] Lacy MK, Nicolau DP, Nightingale CH, Quintiliani R. The pharmacodynamics of aminoglycosides. Clin Infect Dis 1998;27:23–7.
[57] Maderas-Kelly KJ, Ostergaard BE, Hovde LB, Rotschafer JC. Twenty-four-hour area under the concentration-time curve/MIC ratio as a generic predictor or fluoroquinolone antimicrobial effect by using three strains of *Pseudomonas aeruginosa* and an in vitro pharmacodynamic model. Antimicrob Agents Chemother 1996;40:627–32.
[58] Fish DN. Extended-interval dosing of aminoglycoside antibiotics in critically ill patients. J Pharm Pract 2002;15:285–95.
[59] Nicolau DP, McNabb J, Lacy MK, et al. Continuous versus intermittent administration of ceftazidime in intensive care unit patients with nosocomial pneumonia. Int J Antimicrob Agents 2001;17:497–504.
[60] Power BM, Forbes AM, Heerden PV, Ilett KF. Pharmacokinetics of drugs used in critically ill adults. Clin Pharmacokinet 1998;34:25–56.
[61] Leroy O, Jaffre S, d'Escrivan T, et al. Hospital-acquired pneumonia: risk factors for antimicrobial-resistant causative pathogens in critically ill patients. Chest 2003;123:2034–42.
[62] Niederman MS. Use of broad-spectrum antimicrobials for the treatment of pneumonia in seriously ill patients: maximizing clinical outcomes and minimizing selection of resistant organisms. Clin Infect Dis 2006;42(suppl 2):S72–81.
[63] Mouton JW. Combination therapy as a tool to prevent emergence of bacterial resistance. Infection 1999;27(suppl 2):S24–8.
[64] Bouza E, Muñoz P. Monotherapy versus combination therapy for bacterial infections. Med Clin North Am 2000;84:1358–89.
[65] Mouton Y, Debosker Y, Bazin C, et al. Prospective, randomized, controlled study of imipenem-cilastatin versus cefotaxime-amikacin in the treatment of lower respiratory tract infection and septicemia at intensive care units. Presse Med 1990;19:607–12.
[66] Leibovici L, Paul M, Poznanski O, et al. Monotherapy versus beta-lactam-aminoglycoside combination treatment for gram-negative bacteremia: a prospective, observational study. Antimicrob Agents Chemother 1997;41:1127–33.
[67] Hilf M, Yu VL, Sharp J, et al. Antibiotic therapy for *Pseudomonas aeruginosa* bacteremia: outcome correlations in a prospective study of 200 patients. Am J Med 1989;87:540–6.
[68] Chow JW, Fine MJ, Shlaes DM, et al. *Enterobacter* bacteremia: clinical features and emergence of antibiotic resistance during therapy. Ann Intern Med 1991;115:585–90.
[69] Korvick JA, Bryan CS, Farber B, et al. Prospective observational study of *Klebsiella* bacteremia in 230 patients: outcome for antibiotic combinations versus monotherapy. Antimicrob Agents Chemother 1992;36:2639–44.

[70] Vidal F, Mensa J, Almela M, et al. Epidemiology and outcome of *Pseudomonas aeruginosa* bacteremia, with special emphasis on the influence of antibiotic treatment. Arch Intern Med 1996;156:2121–6.
[71] Sigman-Igra Y, Ravona R, Primerman H, Gialdi M. *Pseudomonas aeruginosa* bacteremia: an analysis of 123 episodes, with particular emphasis on the effect of antibiotic therapy. Int J Infect Dis 1998;2:211–5.
[72] Sieger B, Berman SJ, Geckler RW, Farkas SA. Empiric treatment of hospital-acquired lower respiratory tract infections with meropenem or ceftazidime with tobramycin: a randomized study. Crit Care Med 1997;25:1663–70.
[73] Rubinstein E, Lode H, Grassi C. Ceftazidime monotherapy vs. ceftriaxone/tobramycin for serious hospital-acquired gram-negative infections. Antibiotic Study Group. Clin Infect Dis 1995;20:1217–28.
[74] Giantsou E, Liratzopoulos N, Efraimidou E, et al. Both early-onset and late-onset ventilator-associated pneumonia are caused by potentially multiresistant bacteria. Intensive Care Med 2005;31:1488–94.
[75] Burgess DS, Nathisuwan S. Cefepime, piperacillin/tazobactam, gentamicin, ciprofloxacin, and levofloxacin alone and in combination against *Pseudomonas aeruginosa*. Diagn Microbiol Infect Dis 2002;44:35–41.
[76] Fish DN, Choi MK, Jung R. Synergic activity of cephalosporins plus fluoroquinolones against *Pseudomonas aeruginosa* with resistance to one or both drugs. J Antimicrob Chemother 2002; 50:1045–9.
[77] Montravers P, Gauzit R, Muller C, et al. Emergence of antibiotic-resistant bacteria in cases of peritonitis after intra-abdominal surgery affects the efficacy of empirical antimicrobial therapy. Clin Infect Dis 1996;23:486–94.
[78] Singh N, Rogers P, Atwood C, et al. Short-course empiric antibiotic therapy for patients with pulmonary infiltrates in the intensive care unit: a proposed solution for indiscriminate antibiotic prescription. Am J Respir Crit Care Med 2000;162(2 pt 1):505–11.
[79] Chastre J, Wolff M, Fagon J-Y, et al. Comparison of 8 vs. 15 days of antibiotic therapy for ventilator-associated pneumonia in adults: a randomized trial. JAMA 2003;290:2588–98.
[80] Micek ST, Ward S, Fraser VJ, Kollef MH. A randomized controlled trial of an antibiotic discontinuation policy for clinically suspected ventilator-associated pneumonia. Chest 2004;125: 1791–9.
[81] McGowan Jr JE, Gerding DN. Does antibiotic restriction prevent resistance? New Horiz 1996; 4:370–6.
[82] Rice LB, Eckstein EC, DeVente J, Shlaes DM. Ceftazidime-resistant *Klebsiella pneumoniae* isolates recovered at the Cleveland Department of Veterans Affairs Medical Center. Clin Infect Dis 1996;23:118–24.
[83] Giamarellou H, Antoniadou A. The effect of monitoring of antibiotic use on decreasing antibiotic resistance in the hospital. Ciba Found Symp 1997;207:76–86.
[84] Climo MW, Israel DS, Wong ES, et al. Hospital-wide restriction of clindamycin: effect on the incidence of *Clostridium difficile*-associated infection and cost. Ann Intern Med 1998; 128(12 pt 1):989–95.
[85] Burke JP. Antibiotic resistance—squeezing the balloon? JAMA 1998;280:1270–1.
[86] American Thoracic Society, Infectious Diseases Society of America. Guidelines for the management of adults with hospital-acquired, ventilator-associated, and healthcare-associated pneumonia. Am J Respir Crit Care Med 2005;171:388–416.
[87] Rello J, Paiva JA, Baraibar J, et al. International conference for the development of consensus on the diagnosis and treatment of ventilator-associated pneumonia. Chest 2001;120:955–70.
[88] Ibrahim EH, Ward S, Sherman G, et al. Experience with a clinical guideline for the treatment of ventilator-associated pneumonia. Crit Care Med 2001;29:1109–15.
[89] Kollef MH, Vlasnik J, Sharpless L, et al. Scheduled change of antibiotic class: a strategy to decrease the incidence of ventilator-associated pneumonia. Am J Respir Crit Care Med 1997; 156(4 pt 1):1040–8.
[90] Gruson D, Hilbert G, Vargas F, et al. Strategy of antibiotic rotation: long-term effect on incidence

and susceptibilities of Gram-negative bacilli responsible for ventilator-associated pneumonia. Crit Care Med 2003;31:1908–14.
[91] Raymond DP, Pellitier SJ, Crabtree TD, et al. Impact of a rotating empiric antibiotic schedule on infectious mortality in an intensive care unit. Crit Care Med 2001;29:1101–8.
[92] Gruson D, Hilbert G, Vargas F, et al. Rotation and restricted use of antibiotics in a medical intensive care unit: impact on the incidence of ventilator-associated pneumonia caused by antibiotic-resistant Gram-negative bacteria. Am J Respir Crit Care Med 2000;162(3 pt 1): 837–43.
[93] Hughes MG, Evans HL, Chong TW, et al. Effect of an intensive care unit rotating empiric antibiotic schedule on the development of hospital-acquired infections on the non-intensive care unit ward. Crit Care Med 2004;32:53–60.
[94] Regal RE, DePestel DD, VandenBussche HL. The effect of an antimicrobial restriction program on *Pseudomonas aeruginosa* resistance to beta-lactams in a large teaching hospital. Pharmacotherapy 2003;23:618–24.
[95] Paterson DL. The role of antimicrobial management programs in optimizing antibiotic prescribing within hospitals. Clin Infect Dis 2006;42(suppl 2):S90–5.
[96] Gross R, Morgan AS, Kinky DE, et al. Impact of a hospital-based antimicrobial management program on clinical and economic outcomes. Clin Infect Dis 2001;33:289–95.

ELSEVIER
SAUNDERS

Crit Care Clin 22 (2006) 313–327

CRITICAL
CARE
CLINICS

Sedative and Analgesic Medications: Risk Factors for Delirium and Sleep Disturbances in the Critically Ill

Pratik Pandharipande, MD, MSCI[a,*],
E. Wesley Ely, MD, MPH[b,c,d]

[a]*Division of Critical Care, Department of Anesthesiology, Vanderbilt University School of Medicine, 324 MAB, 1313 21st Avenue South, Nashville, TN 37232, USA*
[b]*Department of Medicine, Center for Health Services Research, Vanderbilt University School of Medicine, Nashville, TN 37232, USA*
[c]*Division of Allergy/Pulmonary/Critical Care Medicine, Vanderbilt University School of Medicine, Nashville, TN 37232, USA*
[d]*Center for Health Services Research and the Veterans Administration Tennessee Valley Geriatric Research, Education, and Clinical Center, Nashville, TN 37232, USA*

In an executive summary of medical injury in older patients published by the American Association of Retired Persons (AARP) and the Harvard Schools of Medicine and Public Health [1], acute brain dysfunction (delirium) was considered as one of the six leading causes of preventable injury in those older than 65 years of age. Although physicians in intensive care units (ICUs) are accustomed to recognizing multiple organ dysfunction syndrome (MODS) [2–5], therapy is focused on the causes and treatment of respiratory, cardiovascular, renal, and hepatic dysfunction rather than on delirium. In the past few years, research has shown that the development of delirium during the initial ICU admission is one of the strongest predictors of prolonged cognitive impairment and mortality [6–9]. Hence, interventions aimed at reducing these acute neuro-

P. Pandharipande is a recipient of the Foundation of Anesthesia Education and Research's Mentored Research Grant. E.W. Ely is the Associate Director of Research for the Veterans Administration Tennessee Valley Geriatric Research and Education Clinical Center. He is a recipient of the Paul Beeson Faculty Scholar Award from the Alliance for Aging Research as well as a recipient of a K23 from the National Institutes of Health (grant AG01023-01A1).

* Corresponding author.
E-mail address: pratik.pandharipande@vanderbilt.edu (P. Pandharipande).

doi:10.1016/j.ccc.2006.02.010 ***criticalcare.theclinics.com***

cognitive effects of critical illness are of great importance. The lay public and health care professionals are now becoming increasingly concerned not only with survival but with the preservation of cognitive abilities, prevention of functional decline, and quality of life among patients who survive critical illness [10–14]. In a survey by Fried and colleagues [15], the potential of being left cognitively impaired was the major determinant of patients' treatment preferences at the end of life, with 9 of 10 patients preferring death to severe cognitive impairment. Similarly, in a report from the international "Surviving Intensive Care" 2002 Roundtable Conference held in Brussels [16], the need for future investigations in neurocognitive abnormalities among survivors of intensive care received the strongest recommendation from the international panel of experts. A series of investigations have recently been conducted that provided validated means of detecting delirium by nonpsychiatrists (eg, internists, nurses, respiratory therapists) [17,18]. The central nervous system (CNS) monitoring instruments and observations from these investigations are leading to a change of culture and practice in the ICU, whereby we follow patients more closely for the development of delirium and modify their care to help prevent this potentially disastrous complication.

Delirium: prevalence and subtypes

The prevalence of delirium in medical ICU cohort studies has been reported as 20% [19], 70% [20], or 80% [17] depending on the severity of illness and the delirium detection instrument used. Similarly, delirium is seen in approximately 70% of mechanically ventilated trauma and surgical ICU patients [21]. Its incidence is likely to increase in future years as older persons more frequently receive ICU care. Unfortunately, delirium remains unrecognized by the clinician in as many as 66% to 84% of patients experiencing this complication [22,23], and it may be attributed incorrectly to dementia, depression, or just an "expected" occurrence in the critically ill elderly patient [22]. Peterson and coworkers [24] recently reported on delirium subtypes from a cohort of ventilated and non-ventilated ICU patients in whom delirium was monitored. These investigators found that among patients who developed delirium, pure hyperactive delirium was rare (<5%), whereas hypoactive and mixed types of delirium were the predominant subtypes (~45% each). Interestingly, the hypoactive subtype was significantly more common in older patients than in young patients. The risk factors for and clinical implications of these subtypes are the subject of ongoing investigations.

Prognostic significance of delirium

In non-ICU populations, the development of delirium in the hospital is associated with an in-hospital mortality rate of 25% to 33%, a prolonged hospital stay, and three times the likelihood of discharge to a nursing home [25–27]. In a three-site study of non-ICU medical patients, delirium was found to be an independent predictor of the combined outcome of death or nursing home placement [28]. McCusker and colleagues [29] reported an adjusted hazard of dying of 2.11 associated with the development of delirium. This mortality increase has now been shown to be independent of dementia status [30]. Furthermore, three recent prospective studies found that delirium was associated with an increased risk for dementia over 2 to 3 years [31–33].

Among medical ICU patients, delirium has been shown to be a strong predictor of increased time on mechanical ventilation, longer ICU length of stay, costs, prolonged neuropsychologic dysfunction, and even mortality in two large prospective studies in the medical ICU [6,34,35]. In fact, the development of delirium is associated with a threefold increase in the risk of death after controlling for preexisting comorbidities, severity of illness, coma, and the use of sedative and analgesic medications. These data also showed that delirium is not simply a transition state from coma to normal, because delirium occurred just as often among those who never developed coma as it did among those with coma and persisted in 11% of patients at the time of hospital discharge. This association of delirium with worsening outcomes has recently been shown in a cohort of patients in a trauma and surgical ICU as well [21].

Delirium: pathophysiology

The mechanisms of ICU delirium remain a promising area of study and likely overlap with those leading to long-term cognitive impairment. Long-term cognitive impairment refers to the development of dementia-like symptoms in patients after surviving their critical illness. This has been shown to occur in more than 30% of patients after mechanical ventilation for acute respiratory distress syndrome (ARDS), even a year after their ICU admission [9,36]. From a neuroscience perspective, delirium is thought to be related to imbalances in the synthesis, release, and inactivation of neurotransmitters modulating the control of cognitive function, behavior, and mood [37,38]. Three of the neurotransmitter systems involved in the pathophysiology of delirium are dopamine, gamma-aminobutyric acid (GABA), and acetylcholine [39–41]. Although dopamine increases excitability of neurons, GABA and acetylcholine decrease neuronal excitability [41]. An imbalance in one or more of these neurotransmitters results in neuronal instability and unpredictable neurotransmission. In general, an excess of dopamine and depletion of acetylcholine are two major physiologic problems thought to be central to delirium. In addition to these neurotransmitter systems, others are believed to be involved in the development of delirium, such as serotonin imbalance, endorphin hyperfunction, and increased central noradrenergic activity [38,39]. Other factors thought to be mechanistically deliriogenic in ICU patients include inflammatory abnormalities induced by endotoxin and cytokines, such as tumor necrosis factor (TNF) [42–45]. Cognitive neuroscience and psychopharmacology are active areas of research that may yield advances in our understanding of the pathophysiology of delirium and long-term cognitive impairment.

Risk factors for delirium

Although numerous risk factors for the development of delirium have been identified in non-ICU cohorts [25], only a few studies have examined these in the ICU population. Patients who are highly vulnerable to delirium may develop the disorder after only minor physiologic stressors, whereas those with low baseline vulnerability require a more noxious insult to become delirious [46]. It is possible to stratify patients into risk groups depending on the number of risk factors present [22,46–48]. Three or more risk factors increase the likelihood of developing delirium to approximately 60% or higher, and it is a rare patient in the ICU who would not be in the high-risk group. In an ICU cohort study [49], risk factors related to the medical history included hypertension and smoking. In fact, most ICU patients have more than 10 risk factors for delirium [17,50]. In practical terms, the risk factors can be divided into three categories: (1) host factors, (2) the acute illness itself, and (3) iatrogenic or environmental factors (Table 1). Although delirium may be a function of patients' specific underlying illness, it may also be attributable to medical management issues, and thus preventable causes. Of these risk factors, sedative and analgesic medications and sleep deprivation seem to be the leading iatrogenic, and hence possibly preventable, risk factors for delirium. There are conflicting data on the association of anticholinergics, corticosteroids, histamine-2 antagonists, and anticonvulsants on the development of delirium [22,47,51,52]. Hence, these are not discussed here. The purpose of this article is to review recent data regarding the association of sedatives and analgesic medication with delirium and sleep deprivation, which, in turn, is a risk factor for the development of delirium.

Sedatives and analgesic agents contributing to delirium

Sedative and analgesic medications are routinely administered to patients on mechanical ventilation in accordance with widely recognized clinical practice

Table 1
Selected risk factors for delirium in intensive care unit patients

Host factors	Acute illness	Iatrogenic or environmental
Age	Sepsis[a]	Metabolic disturbances[a]
Baseline comorbidities	Hypoxemia[a]	Anticholinergic medications[a]
Baseline cognitive impairment	Global severity of illness score	Sedative and analgesic medications[a]
Genetic predisposition (?)	Metabolic disturbances[a]	Sleep disturbances[a]

[a] Potentially modifiable factors.

guidelines of the Society of Critical Care Medicine (SCCM) [53] to reduce pain and anxiety. The third component of the clinical practice algorithm published in these same guidelines is delirium. Of pain, anxiety, and delirium (three key components of the guideline's treatment algorithm), only delirium has been determined to be an independent predictor of mortality and ongoing morbidity, such as long-term cognitive impairment. Recent investigations have shown that continuous intravenous sedation is associated with prolonged mechanical ventilation and increased morbidity. Similarly, associations between psychoactive medications and worsening cognitive outcomes have been reported in postsurgical patients. Marcantonio and colleagues [54] performed a nested case-control study within a prospective cohort of postoperative patients who developed delirium and found an association between benzodiazepines and meperidine use and the occurrence of delirium. Dubois and coworkers [49] have shown that opiates (morphine and meperidine) administered intravenously or via an epidural catheter may be associated with the development of delirium in medical or surgical ICU patients. Studies like these have generated concern regarding whether these drugs were actually responsible for the development of delirium or were given as a result of delirium. Our group has recently studied this temporal relation between delirium and the administration of sedatives and analgesics [55]. To do so, one needs to have repeated cognitive assessments and be able to assess the risk factors to which a patient is exposed, in between these assessments, to study which of these factors are associated with a transition or change in cognitive status from normal, delirium, or coma to delirium or normal. We defined patients as normal, delirious, or comatose using well-validated and highly reliable instruments, the Confusion Assessment Method for the ICU (CAM-ICU) [17,18] and the Richmond Agitation-Sedation Scale (RASS) [56,57]. Normal was defined as RASS scores of −3 and higher and CAM-ICU–negative. Delirium was defined as an acute change or fluctuation in mental status accompanied by inattention and disorganized thinking or an altered level of consciousness (RASS scores −3 and higher and CAM-ICU–positive). Coma was defined as a RASS score of −4 or −5, where the CAM-ICU status could not be assessed. The aim of the analysis was to estimate the probability of a transition or change in cognitive status to delirium as a function of sedative and analgesic drug administration in the previous 24 hours and predetermined clinically relevant covariates. Covariates determined a priori after our review of the literature and organized focus group meetings with our ICU staff included age, gender, visual and hearing deficits, history of dementia, depression (measured with the Geriatric Depression Scale short form [58]), severity of illness using the modified Acute Physiology and Chronic Health Evaluation (APACHE II; removing the Glasgow Coma Scale), sepsis, history of neurologic disease, hematocrit (baseline), and daily serum glucose levels. Markov regression modeling (adjusting for 11 covariates mentioned previously) was used in our evaluation of 198 mechanically ventilated patients to determine the probability of daily transition to delirium as a function of sedative and analgesic dose administration over the previous 24 hours. In our study, lorazepam was found to be an independent risk factor for daily transition to delirium (odds ratio [OR] = 1.2, 95% confidence interval [CI], 1.1–1.4); $P = .003$), whereas fentanyl, morphine, and propofol were associated with higher but not statistically significant ORs (Fig. 1) [55]. Increasing age and APACHE II scores were also independent predictors of transitioning to delirium (multivariable $P < .05$) [55]. Similar associations between another benzodiazepine, midazolam, and transition to delirium have been found in a recently completed study in our trauma and surgical ICU patients [21]. The difference represents the sedation practice in our ICUs. Although lorazepam is the drug of choice for anxiolysis and sedation in the medical ICU, midazolam is the agent most frequently used in our trauma and surgical ICUs.

Although it should be emphasized that these medications have an important role in patient comfort, health care professionals must also strive to achieve the right balance of sedative and analgesic administration through greater focus on reducing unnecessary or overzealous use. Instituting daily interruption of sedatives and analgesics or protocolizing their delivery has been shown to improve patients' outcomes [59–61]. Based on the previously mentioned outcome studies [59–61], the SCCM's guidelines [53] recommend that ICU teams of physicians, nurses, and pharmacists set clinically appropriate target sedation levels using well-validated sedation scales. Health care teams should routinely readdress these target levels each day to ensure titration of medications to the desired clinical end point. Unfortunately, no studies to date have measured whether or not such techniques were accompanied by a lower prevalence of delirium. This is surprising, given that these medications affect the CNS; yet, the literature is replete with nonneurologic outcomes of sedative regimens, such as days on me-

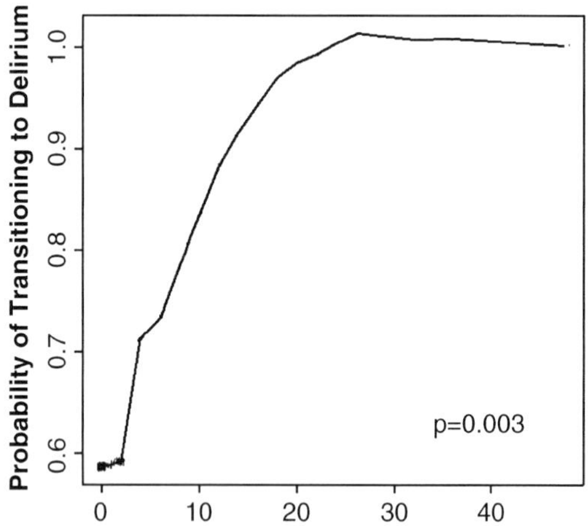

Fig. 1. Lorazepam and the probability of transitioning to delirium. The probability of transitioning to delirium increased with the dose of lorazepam administered in the previous 24 hours. This incremental risk was large at low doses and plateaued at approximately 20 mg/d. (*From* Pandharipande P, Shintani A, Truman Pun B, et al. Lorazepam is an independent risk factor for transitioning to delirium in intensive care unit patients. Anesthesiology 2006;104:23; with permission.)

chanical ventilation, ICU length of stay, and mortality. Ongoing trials are exploring whether changing patterns of sedative and analgesic medication delivery by incorporating mandatory spontaneous breathing trials and/or spontaneous awakening trials affect cognitive outcomes in the critically ill by limiting the exposure to sedatives and analgesics.

It is not clear whether this association of benzodiazepines, and possibly opioids, with delirium is related to the pharmacokinetic properties of the agents or the pharmacodynamics of the drug. Benzodiazepines and propofol have high affinity for the GABA-receptor in the CNS [62]. This GABA-mimetic effect can alter levels of numerous neurotransmitters believed to be deliriogenic [63,64]. Novel sedative agents that are GABA-receptor sparing may help to reduce some of the cognitive dysfunction seen in ICU patients. The approval of α_2-receptor agonists, such as dexmedetomidine, for short-term sedation in the ICU [65] has stimulated research in this area. Recently, Maldonado and colleagues [66] showed in a prospective but nonblind randomized trial that patients undergoing cardiac surgery who were sedated during surgery at sternal closure with dexmedetomidine had a dramatically lower incidence of delirium after surgery (8%) compared with those sedated with propofol (50%) or midazolam (50%). These findings must be confirmed to determine whether differing sedation strategies translate into improved clinical outcomes. Randomized controlled trials are being performed to see if the receptor specificity of sedative medications affects cognitive outcomes in the ICU. A large, prospective, randomized, blind trial is presently underway comparing the prevalence, duration, and severity of delirium in critically ill patients who are sedated with dexmedetomidine or a benzodiazepine.

Critically ill patients are known to have impaired drug-metabolizing enzymes of the liver, such as cytochrome P450 (CYP), which could affect the disposition and pharmacokinetics of the huge doses of sedatives and analgesics that ICU patients nearly universally receive. More than 90% of ventilated patients receive benzodiazepines and opiates [50,67] to improve oxygenation, alleviate anxiety, and prevent removal of support devices. The quantity and dosing intervals are largely empiric and rudimentary, and it is commonplace to find young as well as old patients in a drug-induced coma [68]. Considering the role of age as a susceptibility factor to the development of delirium and long-term cognitive impairment, it is striking that physicians rarely modify the quantity or dosing intervals of these drugs based on patients' age. This flies in the face of evidence that for many drugs, aging results in reduced metabolism [69,70]. It is clear that large doses and extended use of sedatives and analgesics often result in oversedation that may be reduced but not eliminated through the use of clinical target-based sedation protocols [59,60,61,68,71,72]. Whether modification of the dosing regimens and sedation strategies affects the cognitive outcomes of our elderly patients is yet to be studied.

Past studies of the relation between sedatives and analgesics and outcomes have used total drug dose to estimate exposure [22,47,54,73,74]. It has been recognized for more than two decades that drug responses for essentially all

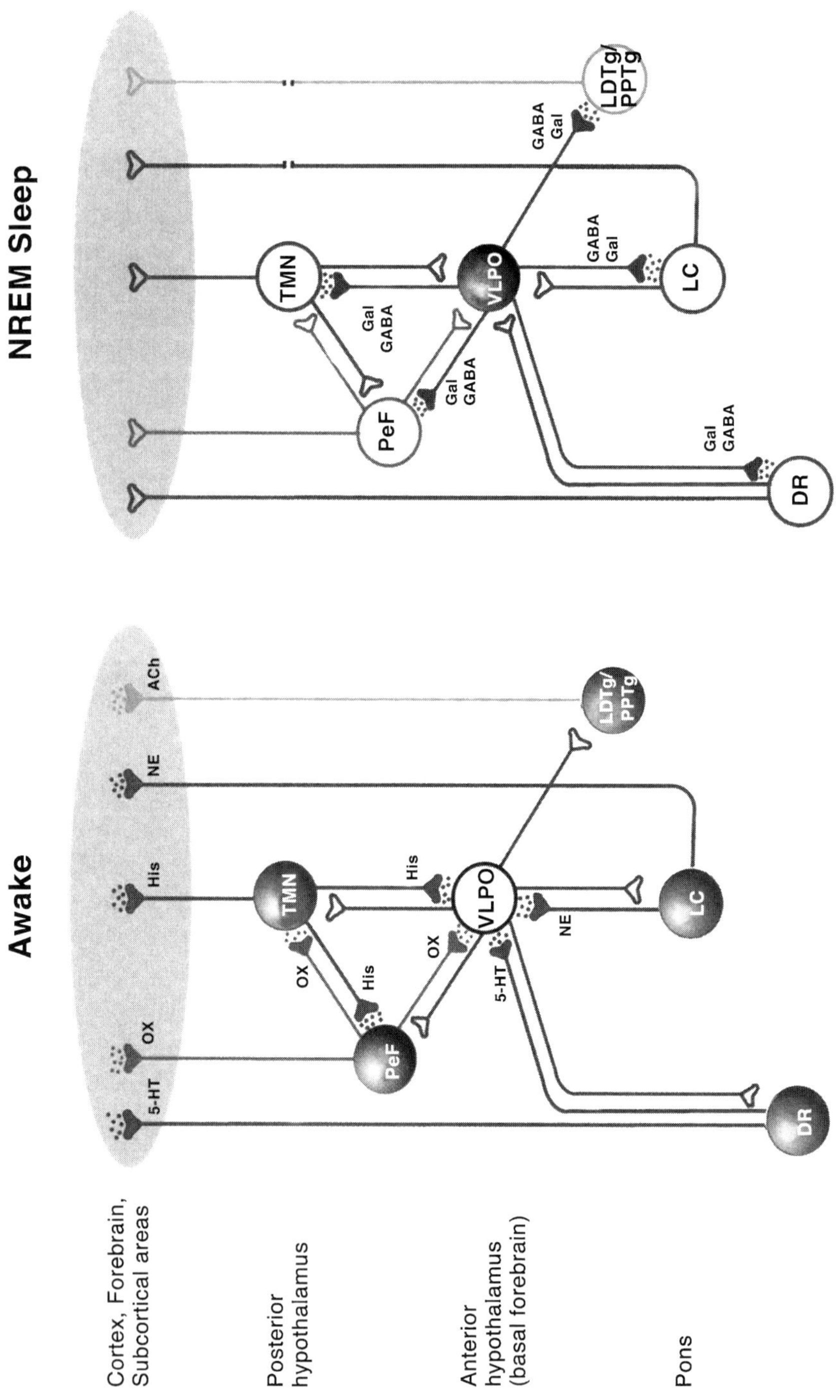
Awake
NREM Sleep
Cortex, Forebrain, Subcortical areas
Posterior hypothalamus
Anterior hypothalamus (basal forebrain)
Pons
5-HT
OX
His
NE
ACh
TMN
PeF
VLPO
LC
DR
LDTg/ PPTg
Gal GABA
GABA Gal

medications exhibit interindividual variability, often marked, when drug dosage alone is considered. This is because the associated drug level leading to a response is determined by the interaction of genetic, environmental, and disease factors modulating drug disposition, including distribution to the brain and other organs. By contrast, there is frequently a better quantitative relation between a drug's plasma concentration and its effects. In healthy volunteers and critically ill patients, for example, a relation exists between levels of sedation induced by short-term midazolam and morphine infusions and their plasma concentrations [75–77]. Accordingly, our understanding of the association between drug exposure and delirium and long-term cognitive impairment may be enhanced by measuring plasma levels of the principal psychoactive drugs to which the patient is exposed. Thus, major questions exist as to the significance of exposure to sedative and analgesic medications in critically ill patients and the development of delirium and long-term cognitive impairment.

Sleep deprivation in the critically ill

The sleep cycle is divided into rapid eye movement (REM) sleep and non–rapid eye movement (NREM) sleep [78]. NREM sleep is further described as stages 1 through 4 depending on increasing depth of sleep [78]. A normal sleep cycle lasts approximately 90 minutes, cycling continuously between REM and NREM sleep. Stages 3 and 4 of NREM sleep represent slow wave or more restful sleep [78].

Critically ill patients have severe sleep deprivation with disruption of sleep architecture. The average amount of sleep in the ICU has been measured to be approximately 2 of 24 hours, with less than 6% of it spent in REM sleep. In a study by Cooper and coworkers [79], most patients had abnormal sleep patterns. The causes of sleep deprivation in the ICU have been extensively reported and consist of excessive noise and lighting; patient care activities, such as procedures and baths; metabolic consequences of critical illness; mechanical ventilation; and sedative and analgesic medications that are administered to these patients [80]. This disturbance in the duration and quality of sleep has detrimental effects on protein synthesis, cellular and humoral immunity, and

---

Fig. 2. Neurotransmitter mechanism for awake fullness and NREM sleep. The VLPO in the anterior hypothalamus is the major area of the brain that controls sleep induction and maintenance. Its major neurotransmitter is GABA, and during the awake state, this GABA release from the VLPO is inhibited by NE from the LC. With the inhibition of GABA, neurotransmitters, such as orexin, serotonin, histamine, and acetylcholine, are released, resulting in a state of wakefulness. During NREM sleep, there is a hierarchic sequence of changes in which inhibition of the LC disinhibits the VLPO to release (GABA and galanin at the projections that terminate at the TMN. These inhibitory neurotransmitters inhibit firing of the TMN projections to the cortical and subcortical regions. ACh, acetylcholine; 5-HT serotonin; His, histamine; LDTg, laterodorsal tegmental nucleus; OX, Orexin; PPTg, pedunculopontine tegmental nucleus; TMN, tuberomammillary nucleus. (*From* Maze M. Analgesics: receptor ligands: alpha 2 adrenergic receptor agonists. In: Bonnet F, editor. Anesthetic pharmacology. Physiologic principles and clinical practice. New York: Elsevier; 2004. p. 477; with permission.)

energy expenditure, resulting in respiratory hemodynamic effects and cognitive function [80,81]. Studies that have looked at sleep disturbances attributable to noise, patient activities, and light have found that only approximately 30% of the sleep arousals were a result of these environmental factors, which suggests that other patient factors or management issues play an important role [82]. Of these, it is interesting that the psychoactive medications are common risk factors for delirium and sleep disturbances, whereas sleep deprivation can itself lead to delirium.

Neurotransmission in sleep

The ventrolateral preoptic nucleus (VLPO) in the anterior hypothalamus is the major area of the brain that controls sleep induction and maintenance [83]. Its major neurotransmitter is GABA, and during the awake state, this GABA release from the VLPO is inhibited by norepinephrine (NE) from the locus ceruleus (LC) [83]. With the inhibition of GABA, neurotransmitters like orexin, serotonin, histamine, and acetylcholine are released, resulting in a state of wakefulness (Fig. 2). During NREM sleep, NE release decreases, thus removing the inhibitory effect on GABA release from the VLPO. With GABA neurons firing, it inhibits the neurotransmitters of wakefulness (orexin, serotonin, histamine, and acetylcholine), resulting in NREM sleep (see Fig. 2). REM sleep, conversely, is facilitated by neurons in the pons, which release acetylcholine. Studies show that serotonin and norepinephrine inhibit these neurons, suppressing REM sleep.

Sedative and analgesic medications are routinely administered to critically ill patients to promote sleep. Although patients seem to be sedated, sleep architecture is often adversely affected [78]. Benzodiazepines and propofol prolong stage 2 NREM sleep while decreasing slow wave sleep and REM sleep. Conversely, opioids increase stage 1 NREM sleep while decreasing slow wave and REM sleep. Numerous other medications routinely administered to critically ill patients affect sleep architecture. These include antiarrhythmic agents, inotropes and vasopressors, antibiotics, antidepressants, steroids, anticonvulsants, and bronchodilators [78]. The effects of these drugs on sleep patterns are summarized in Table 2.

The ω-receptor agonists, such as zolpidem, may preserve REM sleep as well as slow wave sleep, although they lack anxiolytic properties [84]. Similarly, mirtazapine, a noradrenergic and specific serotonergic antidepressant, has been studied in healthy volunteers and shown to improve sleep efficiency while decreasing the number of awakenings and their duration [85]. The slow wave sleep time was also increased, whereas the stage 1 sleep time was decreased significantly. There was no significant effect on REM sleep variables [85]. Recent investigations in rats with dexmedetomidine show that it mimics and increases NREM sleep [83] but decreases REM sleep. By acting on the LC, dexmedetomidine inhibits NE release, thus causing GABA output from the VLPO and inhibition of the neurotransmitters of wakefulness to produce an NREM sleep

Table 2
Drugs commonly used in intensive care unit and their effects on sleep pattern

Drug class or Individual drug	Sleep disorder induced or reported	Possible mechanism
Benzodiazepines	↓ REM, ↓ SWS	Gamma-aminobutyric acid type A receptor stimulation
Opioids	↓ REM, ↓ SWS	μ-receptor stimulation
Clonidine	↓ REM	α_2-receptor stimulation
Nonsteroidal anti-inflammatory drugs	↓ TST, ↓ SE	Prostaglandin synthesis inhibition
Norepinephrine/ epinephrine	Insomnia, ↓ REM, ↓ SWS	α_1-receptor stimulation
Dopamine	Insomnia, ↓ REM, ↓ SWS	D_2 receptor stimulation/α_1-receptor stimulation
β-blockers	Insomnia, ↓ REM, Nightmares	Central nervous system β-blockade by lipophilic agents
Amiodarone	Nightmares	Unknown mechanism
Corticosteroids	Insomnia, ↓ REM, ↓ SWS	Reduced melatonin secretion
Aminophylline	Insomnia, ↓REM, ↓ SWS, ↓ TST, ↓ SE	Adenosine receptor antagonism
Quinolones	Insomnia	Gamma-aminobutyric acid type A receptor inhibition
Tricyclic antidepressants	↓REM	Antimuscarinic activity and α_1-receptor stimulation
Selective serotonin reuptake inhibitors	↓REM, ↓ TST, ↓ SE	Increased serotonergic activity
Phenytoin	↑ Sleep fragmentation	Inhibition of neuronal calcium influx
Phenobarbital	↓ REM	Increased gamma-aminobutyric acid type A activity
Carbamazepine	↓REM	Adenosine receptor stimulation and/or serotonergic activity

Abbreviations: REM, rapid eye movement; SE, sleep efficiency; SWS, slow wave sleep; TST, total sleep time; ↓, decrease; ↑, increase.

pattern. This is in contrast to benzodiazepines and propofol, which exert their sedative action on the VLPO to increase GABA, and decrease the neurotransmitters, such as orexin, histamine, and serotonin. NE release from the LC is not affected, however. Further clinical trials are required to ascertain the role of these medications in improving the quality and quantity of sleep in critically ill patients and to determine if that may help in improving cognitive outcomes in the ICU.

Summary

Sedatives and analgesics are routinely used in critically ill patients, although they have the potential for side effects, such as delirium and sleep architecture disruption. Although it should be emphasized that these medications are extremely important in providing patient comfort, health care professionals must also strive to achieve the right balance of sedative and analgesic administration through greater focus on reducing unnecessary or overzealous use. Ongoing clinical trials should help us to understand whether altering the delivery strategy, via daily sedation interruption, or protocolized target-based sedation or changing sedation paradigms to target different CNS receptors can affect cognitive outcomes and sleep preservation in our critically ill patients.

References

[1] Rothschild JM, Leape LL, Smith AH. The nature of extent of medical injury in older patients—executive summary. American Association of Retired Persons (AARP) Public Policy Institute Issue Paper #2000-17:2000.

[2] Bone RC. Multiple system organ failure and the sepsis syndrome. Hosp Pract 1991;26:101–9.

[3] Bone RC. Sepsis, the sepsis syndrome, multiorgan failure: a plea for comparable definitions. Ann Intern Med 1991;114:332–3.

[4] Bone RC, Grodzin CJ, Balk RA. Sepsis: a new hypothesis for pathogenesis of the disease process. Chest 1997;112:235–43.

[5] Russell JA, Singer J, Bernard G, et al. Changing pattern of organ dysfunction in early human sepsis is related to mortality. Crit Care Med 2000;28:3405–11.

[6] Ely EW, Shintani A, Truman B, et al. Delirium as a predictor of mortality in mechanically ventilated patients in the intensive care unit. JAMA 2004;291:1753–62.

[7] Hopkins RO, Weaver LK, Pope D, et al. Neuropsychological sequelae and impaired health status in survivors of severe acute respiratory distress syndrome. Am J Respir Crit Care Med 1999;160:50–6.

[8] Jackson JC, Gordon SM, Hart RP, et al. The association between delirium and cognitive decline: a review of the empirical literature. Neuropsychol Rev 2004;14(2):87–98.

[9] Jackson JC, Hart RP, Gordon SM, et al. Six-month neuropsychological outcome of medical intensive care unit patients. Crit Care Med 2003;31:1226–34.

[10] Comarow A. You're never too old. Surgery on patients of 80, 90, and up? It's gaining acceptance. US News World Rep 2004;137(1):83–8.

[11] Inouye SK, Bogardus ST, Baker DI, et al. The hospital elder life program: a model of care to prevent cognitive and functional decline in older hospitalized patients. J Am Geriatr Soc 2000;48:1697–706.

[12] Inouye SK, Peduzzi PN, Robison JT, et al. Importance of functional measures in predicting mortality among older hospitalized patients. JAMA 1998;279(15):1187–93.

[13] Mehta KM, Yaffe K, Covinsky KE. Cognitive impairment, depressive symptoms, and functional decline in older people. J Am Geriatr Soc 2002;50:1045–50.

[14] National Research Council. The aging mind: Opportunities in cognitive research. In: Stern PC, Carstensen LL, editors. 1st edition. Washington, (DC): National Academy Press; 2000. p. 1–249.

[15] Fried TR, Bradley EH, Towle VR, et al. Understanding the treatment preferences of seriously ill patients. N Engl J Med 2002;346:1061–6.

[16] Angus DC, Carlet J. Surviving intensive care: a report from the 2002 Brussels Roundtable. Intensive Care Med 2003;293:366–77.

[17] Ely EW, Inouye SK, Bernard GR, et al. Delirium in mechanically ventilated patients: validity and reliability of the confusion assessment method for the intensive care unit (CAM-ICU). JAMA 2001;286:2703–10.

[18] Ely EW, Margolin R, Francis J, et al. Evaluation of delirium in critically ill patients: validation of the confusion assessment method for the intensive care unit (CAM-ICU). Crit Care Med 2001;29:1370–9.

[19] Bergeron N, Dubois MJ, Dumont M, et al. Intensive Care Delirium Screening Checklist: evaluation of a new screening tool. Intensive Care Med 2001;27:859–64.

[20] McNicoll L, Pisani MA, Zhang Y, et al. Delirium in the intensive care unit: occurrence and clinical course in older patients. J Am Geriatr Soc 2003;51:591–8.
[21] Pandharipande P, Cotton B, Costabile S, et al. Prevalence of delirium in the surgical ICU. Crit Care 2005;33(12):A45.
[22] Francis J, Martin D, Kapoor WN. A prospective study of delirium in hospitalized elderly. JAMA 1990;263:1097–101.
[23] Inouye SK. The dilemma of delirium: clinical and research controversies regarding diagnosis and evaluation of delirium in hospitalized elderly medical patients. Am J Med 1994;97:278–88.
[24] Peterson JF, Truman BL, Shintani A, et al. The prevalence of hypoactive, hyperactive, and mixed type delirium in medical ICU patients. J Am Geriatr Soc 2003;51(Suppl):S174.
[25] American Psychiatric Association. Practice guideline for the treatment of patients with delirium. Am J Psychiatry 1999;156(Suppl):1–20.
[26] Inouye SK, Schlesinger MJ, Lyndon TJ. Delirium: a symptom of how hospital care is failing older persons and a window to improve quality of hospital care. Am J Med 1999;106:565–73.
[27] Levkoff SE, Evans DA, Liptzin B, et al. Delirium: the occurrence and persistence of symptoms among elderly hospitalized patients. Arch Intern Med 1992;152:334–40.
[28] Inouye SK, Rushing JT, Foreman MD, et al. Does delirium contribute to poor hospital outcomes? A three-site epidemiologic study. J Gen Intern Med 1998;13:234–42.
[29] McCusker J, Cole M, Abrahamowicz M, et al. Delirium predicts 12 month mortality. Arch Intern Med 2002;162:457–63.
[30] Fick DM, Agostini JV, Inouye SK. Delirium superimposed on dementia: a systematic review. JAGS 2002;50:1723–32.
[31] McCusker J, Cole M, Dendukuri N, et al. Delirium in older medical inpatients and subsequent cognitive and functional status: a prospective study. Can Med Assoc J 2001;165:575–83.
[32] Rahkonen T, Luukkainen-Markkula R, Paanilla S, et al. Delirium episode as a sign of undetected dementia among community dwelling subjects: a 2 year follow up study. J Neurol Neurosurg Psychiatry 2000;69:519–21.
[33] Rockwood K, Cosway S, Carver D. The risk of dementia and death after delirium. Age Ageing 1999;28(6):551–6.
[34] Lin SM, Liu CY, Wang CH, et al. The impact of delirium on the survival of mechanically ventilated patients. Crit Care Med 2004;32:2254–9.
[35] Milbrandt E, Deppen S, Harrison P, et al. Costs associated with delirium in mechanically ventilated patients. Crit Care Med 2004;32:955–62.
[36] Hopkins RO, Collingridge D, Weaver LK, et al. Neuropsychological sequelae following acute respiratory distress syndrome: two year outcome. J Int Neuropsychol Soc 2003;9:584.
[37] Justic M. Does "ICU psychosis" really exist? Crit Care Nurse 2000;20:28–37.
[38] Meagher DJ, Trzepacz PT. Motoric subtypes of delirium. Semin Clin Neuropsychiatry 2000;5:75–85.
[39] Crippen D. Treatment of agitation and its comorbidities in the intensive care unit. In: Hill NS, Levy MM, editors. Ventilator management strategies for critical care (lung biology in health and disease). New York: Marcel Dekker; 2001. p. 243–84.
[40] Pavlov VA, Wang H, Czura CJ, et al. The cholinergic anti-inflammatory pathway: a missing link in neuroimmunomodulation. Mol Med 2003;9(5–8):125–34.
[41] Webb JM, Carlton EF, Geeham DM. Delirium in the intensive care unit: are we helping the patient? Critical Care Nurs Q 2000;22(4):47–60.
[42] Arvin B, Neville LF, Barone FC, et al. Brain injury and inflammation: a putative role for TNF-alpha. Ann NY Acad Sci 1995;116:62–71.
[43] Bellingan G. The pulmonary physician in critical care—6: the pathogenesis of ALI/ARDS. Thorax 2002;57:540–6.
[44] Fink MP, Evans TW. Mechanisms of organ dysfunction in critical illness: report from a round table conference held in Brussels. Intensive Care Med 2002;28:369–75.
[45] Fulkerson W, MacIntyre N, Stamler J, et al. Pathogenesis and treatment of the adult respiratory distress syndrome. Arch Intern Med 1996;156:29–38.

[46] Inouye SK, Charpentier PA. Precipitating factors for delirium in hospitalized elderly persons: predictive model and interrelationship with baseline vulnerability. JAMA 1996;275: 852–7.
[47] Inouye SK, Viscoli C, Horwitz RI, et al. A predictive model for delirium in hospitalized elderly medical patients based on admission characteristics. Ann Intern Med 1993;119:474–81.
[48] Marcantonio ER, Goldman L, Mangione CM, et al. A clinical prediction rule for delirium after elective noncardiac surgery. JAMA 1994;271:134–9.
[49] Dubois MJ, Bergeron N, Dumont M, et al. Delirium in an intensive care unit: a study of risk factors. Intensive Care Med 2001;27:1297–304.
[50] Ely EW, Gautam S, Margolin R, et al. The impact of delirium in the intensive care unit on hospital length of stay. Intensive Care Med 2001;27:1892–900.
[51] Francis J, Kapoor WN. Delirium in hospitalized elderly. J Gen Intern Med 1990;5:65–79.
[52] Lipowski ZJ. Delirium in the elderly patient. N Engl J Med 1989;320:578–82.
[53] Jacobi J, Fraser GL, Coursin DB, et al. Clinical practice guidelines for the sustained use of sedatives and analgesics in the critically ill adult. Crit Care Med 2002;30:119–41.
[54] Marcantonio ER, Juarez G, Goldman L, et al. The relationship of postoperative delirium with psychoactive medications. JAMA 1994;272:1518–22.
[55] Pandharipande P, Shintani A, Truman Pun B, et al. Lorazepam is an independent risk factor for transitioning to delirium in intensive care unit patients. Anesthesiology 2006;104:21–6.
[56] Ely EW, Truman B, Shintani A, et al. Monitoring sedation status over time in ICU patients: reliability and validity of the Richmond Agitation-Sedation Scale (RASS). JAMA 2003;289: 2983–91.
[57] Sessler CN, Gosnell M, Grap MJ, et al. The Richmond Agitation-Sedation Scale: validity and reliability in adult intensive care patients. Am J Respir Crit Care Med 2002;166:1338–44.
[58] Sheikh JL, Yesavage JA. Geriatric Depression Scale (GDS): recent evidence and development of a shorter version. Clin Gerontol 1986;5:165–73.
[59] Brook AD, Ahrens TS, Schaiff R, et al. Effect of a nursing implemented sedation protocol on the duration of mechanical ventilation. Crit Care Med 1999;27:2609–15.
[60] Kollef MH, Levy NT, Ahrens T, et al. The use of continuous IV sedation is associated with prolongation of mechanical ventilation. Chest 1999;114:541–8.
[61] Kress JP, Pohlman AS, O'Connor MF, et al. Daily interruption of sedative infusions in critically ill patients undergoing mechanical ventilation. N Engl J Med 2000;342:1471–7.
[62] Mihic S, Harris R. GABA and the GABAA receptor. Alcohol Health Res World 1997;21: 127–31.
[63] Van Der Mast RC. Delirium: the underlying pathophysiological mechanisms and the need for clinical research. J Psychosom Res 1996;41:109–13.
[64] Van Der Mast RC. Pathophysiology of delirium. J Geriatr Psychiatry Neurol 1998;11(3): 138–45.
[65] Maze M, Scarfini C, Cavaliere F. New agents for sedation in the intensive care unit. Crit Care Clin 2001;17:881–97.
[66] Maldonado JR, van der Starre PJ, Wysong A. Post-operative sedation and the incidence of ICU delirium in cardiac surgery patients. ASA meeting abstracts. Anesthesiology 2003;99:465.
[67] Esteban A, Anzueto A, Frutos F, et al. Characteristics and outcomes in adult patients receiving mechanical ventilation: a 28-day international study. JAMA 2002;287:345–55.
[68] Heffner JE. A wake-up call in the intensive care unit. N Engl J Med 2000;342:1520–2.
[69] Greenblatt DJ, Harmatz JS, Shader RI. Clinical pharmacokinetics of anxiolytics and hypnotics in the elderly. Therapeutic considerations (part I). Clin Pharmacokinet 1991;21(3):165–77.
[70] Greenblatt DJ, Harmatz JS, Shader RI. Clinical pharmacokinetics of anxiolytics and hypnotics in the elderly. Therapeutic considerations (part II). Clin Pharmacokinet 1991;21(4): 262–73.
[71] Ely EW, O'Meade M, Haponik E, et al. Mechanical ventilator weaning protocols driven by non-physician health care professionals. Chest 2001;120(Suppl):454S–63S.

[72] MacIntyre NR, Cook DJ, Ely EW, et al. Evidence-based guidelines for weaning and discontinuing ventilatory support. Chest 2001;120:375S–95S.
[73] American Psychiatric Association. Delirium, dementia and amnestic and other cognitive disorders. Diagnostic and statistical manual of mental disorders. Arlington (VA): American Psychiatric Publishing, Inc.; 1994. p. 123–33.
[74] Moller J, Cluitmans P, Rasmussen L, et al. Long-term postoperative cognitive dysfunction in the elderly: ISPOCD1 study (International Study of Postoperative Cognitive Dysfunction investigators). Lancet 1998;351:857–61.
[75] Dershwitz M, Walsh JL, Morishige RJ, et al. Pharmacokinetics and pharmacodynamics of inhaled versus intravenous morphine in healthy volunteers. Anesthesiology 2000;93:619–28.
[76] Sarton E, Olofsen E, Romberg R, et al. Sex differences in morphine analgesia: an experimental study in healthy volunteers. Anesthesiology 2000;93:1245–54.
[77] Somma J, Donner A, Zomorodi K, et al. Population pharmacodynamics of midazolam administered by target controlled infusion in SICU patients after CABG surgery. Anesthesiology 1998; 89:1430–43.
[78] Bourne RS, Mills GH. Sleep disruption in critically ill patients—pharmacological considerations. Anaesthesia 2004;59(4):374–84.
[79] Cooper AB, Thornley KS, Young GB, et al. Sleep in critical ill patients requiring mechanical ventilation. Chest 2000;117:809–18.
[80] Gabor JY, Cooper AB, Crombach SA, et al. Contribution of the intensive care unit environment to sleep disruption in mechanically ventilated patients and health subjects. Am J Respir Crit Care Med 2003;167:708–15.
[81] Helton MC, Gordon SH, Nunnery SL. The correlation between sleep deprivation and the intensive care unit syndrome. Heart Lung 1980;9:464–8.
[82] Freedman NS, Gazendam J, Levan L, et al. Abnormal sleep/wake cycles and the effect of environmental noise on sleep disruption in the intensive care unit. Am J Respir Crit Care Med 2001;163:451–7.
[83] Nelson LE, Lu J, Guo T, et al. The a_2-adrenoceptor agonist dexmedetomidine converges on an endogenous sleep-promoting pathway to exert its sedative effects. Anesthesiology 2003;98: 428–36.
[84] Langtry HD, Benfield P. Zolpidem. A review of its pharmacodynamic and pharmacokinetic properties and therapeutic potential. Drugs 1990;40(2):291–313.
[85] Aslan S, Isik E, Cosar B. The effects of mirtazapine on sleep: a placebo controlled, double-blind study in young healthy volunteers. Sleep 2002;25(6):677–9.

ELSEVIER
SAUNDERS

Crit Care Clin 22 (2006) 329–345

CRITICAL
CARE
CLINICS

Drug-Associated Disease: Cytochrome P450 Interactions

Henry J. Mann, PharmD

Department of Experimental and Clinical Pharmacology, College of Pharmacy, University of Minnesota, 7-153 WDH, 308 Harvard Street SE, Minneapolis, MN 55455, USA

The number of reports of drug interactions is so great as to be overwhelming to most clinicians. On average over the last decade there were 60 papers per year cited in PubMed with "drug interaction" in the title, and 1420 papers had drug interaction as a MeSH Major Topic [1]. Most of these publications are not human trials, and only a small number was conducted in specific patient populations. Because of the wide therapeutic index of most marketed drugs, most drug interactions do not cause harm to patients, and some are even used therapeutically. These drug interactions may be a result of physical and chemical interactions (alterations in pH, ionic complexation), competition for pharmacokinetic processes (interference with membrane transport proteins and enzymatic processes involved with intestinal absorption, metabolism, and renal excretion), or they may be pharmacodynamic in nature (competitive inhibition at receptor sites, augmenting receptor stimulation) [2]. This article focuses on the drug interactions that are likely to cause harm in critically ill patients and that are mediated through the cytochrome P450 enzyme system (CYP450). Critical care practitioners should understand the mechanism that underlies the drug interactions that are likely to occur with the medications that are used commonly in critical illness. Also, critical care practitioners must have access to accurate and timely drug interaction resources in their work environment. Generally, such resources are a combination of computer programs, Internet sites, and compendia.

Drug interactions are a specific type of adverse drug effect that usually are predictable, if not preventable. The contribution of drug interactions to overall

E-mail address: hmann@umn.edu

doi:10.1016/j.ccc.2006.02.004 *criticalcare.theclinics.com*

adverse drug effects is significant in terms of incidence and financial cost. The incidence of drug interactions may be increasing as a result of the increased use of medications in the elderly, increasingly complex treatment approaches to common disease states, and increased awareness of adverse drug reactions. In addition to the elderly and patients who take multiple drugs, patients who have renal or liver disease are at an increased risk for drug interactions [3].

The outcome of drug interactions has been reported rarely; most interactions are theoretic and only pose potential adverse effects. When outcomes have been evaluated the cost and morbidity have been significant [4–7]. A recent cost analysis of decreasing the interaction between warfarin and nonsteroidal anti-inflammatory drugs (NSAIDs) through the use of cyclooxygenase (COX)-2–selective NSAIDs proposed an overall health care savings that was due to the decrease in bleeding rate [8]. The impact of drug interactions on the pharmaceutical industry also is significant. Of the 548 drugs that were introduced between 1975 and 1999, 56 (10.2%) had new drug–drug interaction warnings in their package inserts (or label), or were withdrawn from the market for these reasons [9]. Half of those withdrawals occurred after the products had been on the market for more than 7 years, and millions of patient exposures had occurred. Between 1997 and 2000 four drugs (terfenadine, astemizole, cisapride, mibefradil) that are metabolized by the CYP450 system—and subject to drug–drug interactions that increased the likelihood of arrhythmias because of prolongation of the QT interval—were removed from the United States market. Given the tremendous cost of research and development to bring a new drug to market (~$802 million in 2000), the loss of such a product from the market is significant [10]. One of the approaches that the industry has taken to decrease the likelihood of having to drop a drug from development because of drug interactions is to screen candidate drugs for CYP450 interactions at the preclinical stage [11,12]. There are multiple problems in projecting the results of in vitro testing to the clinical situation. Current drug interaction screening can only indicate that a compound's likelihood of drug interaction is "highly possible" or "least likely" [13–18].

The US Food and Drug Administration (FDA) guidance for industry has been published for the conduct of in vitro and in vivo drug metabolism and drug interaction studies, and this information is now expected to be included in the package insert [19–21]. The number of in vivo drug interaction studies that were conducted on new drug applications submitted to the FDA was increasing before the publication of the guidance document. During the period of 1987 to 1991, only 30% of new drug applications had an in vivo drug interaction study, whereas during the period of 1992 to 1997 this percentage was 53% [22]. Most (62%) of the drug interaction studies that were conducted during this period suggested less than a 20% change in some measured pharmacokinetic parameter; 24% were deemed not clinically significant and 14% resulted in a labeling change. One percent resulted in a recommendation for monitoring, and 4% resulted in a labeled contraindication.

Overview of cytochrome P450 isozymes in drug metabolism

The CYP450 enzymes are a superfamily of heme-containing, microsomal drug-metabolizing enzymes that are important in the biosynthesis and degradation of endogenous compounds, chemicals, toxins, and medications. More than 2700 individual members of the CYP450 superfamily have been identified, and 57 cytochrome P enzymes are recognized in man [23]. They perform a variety of chemical processes that lead to the oxidation, reduction, and hydrolysis of substrates to make them more water soluble, which facilitates elimination. Drugs that have undergone biotransformation by the CYP450 enzymes may be activated from a prodrug, converted to an active metabolite, or metabolized to an inactive form. During this phase 1 reaction process the drug substrate is transformed by addition of conversion of a functional group, such as a hydroxyl, amine, or sulfhydryl [24]. Products of the phase 1 reaction may be excreted or metabolized further by synthetic and conjugation reactions (phase 2 reactions) that combine endogenous substances (eg, glucuronic acid, glutathione, sulfur, glycine) with the new functional group [25]. Following phase 2 reactions, metabolites usually are extremely polar and are excreted readily in the urine. The same processes that metabolize exogenous drugs and toxins also synthesize or degrade endogenous substances, such as steroid hormones, cholesterol, eicosanoids, and bile acids. Thus, there is a constant competition for the activity of these enzyme systems which can lead to drug–drug interactions, drug–disease interactions, drug–herbal interactions, and drug–food interactions.

The cytochrome P450 isozymes

CYP3A4 is the CYP450 isozyme that is involved most frequently in drug metabolism. The nomenclature for these enzymes is as follows: CYP represents the root symbol for all cytochrome P450 proteins; 3 denotes the gene family; A designates the subfamily; and 4 represents the individual gene. CYP450 proteins with more than 40% amino acid sequence identity are included in the same family; mammalian sequences with greater than 55% identity are included in the same subfamily. The gene families CYP1, CYP2, and CYP3 are involved largely in biotransformation of drugs, whereas the remaining 15 families in humans perform endogenous metabolic activities (Table 1) [23,26]. CYP3A4 and CYP3A5 account for the metabolism of approximately 50% of marketed drugs, and they make up approximately 60% of the total hepatic CYP450 enzyme content [27–29]. The metabolism of more than 90% of the most clinically important medications can be accounted for by seven cytochrome P (CYP) isozymes (3A4, 3A5, 1A2, 2C9, 2C19, 2D6, and 2E1) [30].

The CYP2 family is the largest in humans and contains about one third of human CYP450 enzymes. The CYP2 family has multiple polymorphisms that can result in decreased enzyme activity or enhanced enzyme activity, which lead to patients being categorized into three unique phenotypes: poor metabolizers,

Table 1
Cytochrome P450 subfamilies and functions in humans

Cytochrome P family	Subfamilies	Function
1	A1, A2, B1	Drug metabolism
2	A6, A13, B6, C8, C9, C18, C19, D6, E1, F1, J2	Drug and steroid metabolism
3	A4, A5, A7, A43	Drug metabolism
4	A11, B1, F2, F3, F8, F12	Arachidonic acid and fatty acid metabolism
5	A1	Thromboxane synthase
7	A1, B1	Steroid 7-α-hydroxylase
8	A1, B1	Bile acid biosynthesis and prostacyclin synthase
11	A1, B1, B2	Steroid biosynthesis
17	A1	Steroid biosynthesis (steroid 17-α-hydroxylase)
19	A1	Steroid biosynthesis (aromatase)
20	A1	Unknown
21	A1	Steroid biosynthesis
24	A1	Vitamin D deactivation
26	A1	Retinoic acid hydroxylase
27	A1	Bile acid biosynthesis and vitamin D3 activation
39	A1	Unknown
46	A1	Cholesterol 24-hydroxylase
51	A1	Lanosterol 14-α-demethylase

Data from Lewis DF. 57 varieties: the human cytochromes P450. Pharmacogenomics 2004;5:305–18; and Danielson PB. The cytochrome P450 superfamily: biochemistry, evolution and drug metabolism in humans. Curr Drug Metab 2002;3:561–97.

extensive metabolizers, and ultrarapid metabolizers [31]. The importance of identifying a patient's phenotype is in its infancy, but a system is being marketed that will determine the genotype of a patient's CYP2D6 or CYP2C19 (AmpliChip CYP450; Roche Molecular Systems, Inc., Pleasanton, California) [32]. When drugs have a narrow therapeutic index and are metabolized primarily by a single CYP isozyme they present a greater risk for problems in patients with poor or ultrarapid metabolism phenotypes. Poor metabolizers have higher concentrations of drug in their bodies, whereas ultrarapid metabolizers may have subtherapeutic concentrations with normal dosing. There are ethnic differences in the frequency of these phenotypes in the population [33,34].

The CYP isozymes are under genetic control and can be expressed to a varying degree in each individual [35,36]. Multiple factors, such as smoking, ethanol consumption, environmental factors, disease states, and genetic inheritance, influence the amount and the activity of an individual patient's CYP isozymes (Table 2) [11,30,37]. Patients who have cirrhotic liver disease primarily have decreased drug metabolizing capability because of a decreased amount of liver tissue, and all of the CYP isozymes are affected [38,39]. The degree to which individual CYPs are reduced is not uniform, however, because CYP1A, 2C, and 3A are more affected than others [40,41]. CYPs also are down-regulated during inflammation and infection, which may lead to these patients being more susceptible to adverse effects and drug interactions [42].

Table 2
Cytochrome P450 isozymes

Cytochrome P isoenzyme	Percent of total CYP	Variability	Percent of drugs metabolized	Activity influenced by
1A1,2	~13	~40 fold	13	Genetic polymorphism; nutrition; smoking; drugs; environmental xenobiotics
1B1	<1		1	Environmental xenobiotics
2A6	~4	~100 fold	3	Genetic polymorphism; drugs; environmental xenobiotics
2B6	<1	~50 fold	4	Drugs
2C9,19	~18	~100 fold	35	Genetic polymorphism; drugs
2D6	Up to 2.5	>1000 fold	15	Genetic polymorphism; drugs
2E1	Up to 7	~20 fold	3	Genetic polymorphism; nutrition; alcohol; environmental xenobiotics
3A4,5	Up to 28	~20 fold	36	Nutrition; drugs; environmental xenobiotics

Data from Refs. [11,30,37].

The CYP450 enzymatic metabolism of a drug (or substrate) can be blocked or inhibited by another drug or it can be accelerated when the enzyme system is induced. Inhibition can be temporary and concentration dependent or it can be the result of a permanent interference with the enzyme; drugs that cause the inhibition are referred to as reversible and irreversible (mechanism-based or suicide) inhibitors [43]. The most common type of drug interaction is simple competitive inhibition for the enzyme reactive site. With simple competitive inhibition the dosing intervals of the interacting drugs can be manipulated to decrease the extent of the interaction when coadministration is required. When irreversible inhibition occurs, a metabolic intermediate is formed by the permanent binding of the inhibiting drug with the P450 enzyme at the heme, the protein, or both. Irreversible inhibitors are of particular importance because they can decrease the first pass clearance and the functional catalytic activity of drugs that normally are cleared by CYP3A4 until new enzyme can be manufactured [43]. Examples of commonly used irreversible inhibitors of CYP3A4 are clarithromycin, erythromycin, isoniazid, carbamazepine, irinotecan, tamoxifen, ritonavir, verapamil, nicardipine, 17-α-ethynylestradiol, fluoxetine, midazolam, and products in grapefruit juice (bergamottin, 6′7′-dihydroxybergamottin) [43].

Many drugs can be substrates for multiple cytochrome P isozymes as well as inducers or inhibitors of multiple cytochrome P isozymes [44]. Table 3 contains some common drugs that are used in ICUs, and the cytochrome isozymes for which they are substrates, inhibitors, and inducers [44–46].

Clinically significant drug interactions

With more than 100,000 drug–drug interactions being documented, distinguishing those of clinical importance is mandatory [47–53]. A drug interaction

Table 3
Frequent substrates, inhibitors, and inducers of P450 isozymes in critically ill patients

Drug	Substrate	Inhibitor	Inducer
Acetaminophen	1A2, 2E1		
Amiodarone		2C9, 2D6, 3A	
Cimetidine		1A2, 2C19, 2D6, 3A	
Codeine	2D6		
Conivaptan	3A4	3A4	
Diltiazem	3A	3A	
Fluconazole		2C9	
Fluoroquinolones		1A2	
Haloperidol	2D6, 3A	2D6	
Halothane	2E1		
Hydrocortisone	3A		3A
Ibuprofen	2C9		
Insulin			1A2
Lidocaine	2D6, 3A		
Methadone		2D6	
Metoprolol	2D6		
Metronidazole		2C9, 3A	
Nafcillin			1A2
Omeprazole	2C19	2C19	1A2
Ondansetron	2D6		
Pantoprazole	2C19, 3A4		
Phenobarbital			2B6, 3A
Phenytoin	2C19, 2C9		2B6, 3A
Prednisone			2C19
Ranitidine		2D6	
Rifampin			2B6, 2C8, 2C19, 2C9, 2D6, 3A
Sildenafil	3A		
Sulfamethoxazole		2C9	
Tacrolimus	3A		
Tamoxifen	2D6, 3A4		
Theophylline	1A2, 2E1		
Trimethoprim		2C8, 2C9	
Warfarin	2C9		

Data from Refs. [44–46].

can be significant because it results in some grievous consequence to the patient or because of its common nature, many patients are exposed to possible harm. Fortunately, most drug interactions do not fall into these two categories. Nonetheless, most pharmacy computer drug interaction software is sensitive to many interactions, regardless of severity. The pharmacist and other clinicians can tend to become accustomed to the routine interaction alarms that are of little clinical significance, and miss or ignore the truly significant alarms that signify real harm [54].

The difference between potential drug interactions and significant drug interactions is illustrated by a recent study from Denmark [55]. A total of 200 medical and surgical patients who were discharged from a hospital were surveyed and visited to ascertain the medications that they had in their homes and how frequently they used them. This information was cross-referenced with a drug-interaction database and with hospital records to clarify the impact of the possible interactions. The average age of patients was 75 years; the median number of drugs used was 8 (range, 1–24 drugs). Drug usage consisted of prescription medications (93% of patients), over-the-counter medications (91% of patients), and herbal medications or dietary supplements (63% of patients). A total of 476 potential drug interactions was identified in 63% of the patients. None of the interactions represented absolute contraindications to the use of the interacting drugs together. Only 21 (4.4%) were classified as relative contraindications [56]. As the number of medications that a patient was taking increased, the risk for potential drug interactions also increased. Patients who were taking 3 to 5 drugs had a 29% risk for potential interaction, and patients who were taking 11 or more drugs had a 96% risk for having a potential drug interaction. None of the potential drug interactions actually resulted in an adverse event based on a review of the patients' charts. Although 65% of patients knew the purpose for each medication that they were prescribed, only 1% of patients were aware of the potential for a drug–drug or drug–food interaction. Previous reports showed that potential drug interactions actually translate to adverse events in 0% to 24% of patients [55,57–59].

To address the problems with identifying clinically significant drug interactions and reducing their occurrence, a Partnership to Prevent Drug-Drug Interactions (PP-DDI) was formed recently. PP-DDI performed an analysis of commonly occurring drug interactions in ambulatory patients, and narrowed the number of clinically important interactions to 25 through careful evaluation of the literature and ratings by an expert panel using a modified Delphi process [60]. The correlation of four common drug interaction compendia on interaction or severity also was evaluated during the study [61]. Drug interactions were rated on a scale of code 1: highly clinically significant; code 2: moderately clinically significant; code 3: minimally clinically significant; and code 4: not clinically significant. Ratings were based on potential harm to the patient, frequency and predictability of occurrence, and degree and quality of documentation. A total of 406 drug interactions were listed at the highest level of severity (code 1) by at least one of the four references. Poor agreement between the references was observed. Only 9 (2.2%) interactions were rated as code 1 in all four compendia, and another 35 (8.6%) were rated code 1 by three of the compendia. Most interactions (71.7%) were listed as most severe in only one reference. Although not yet studied, one would expect similar findings in hospitalized patients.

The frequency of occurrence for the 25 clinically significant drug interactions that were identified by the PP-DDI was studied using a large pharmacy benefit management company (PBM) database [62]. The study found that 374,000 of 46 million plan participants potentially were exposed to one of the 25 clinically significant drug interactions over a 25-month period. Notification of these interactions were sent to the pharmacy where the prescription was being filled; however, in two thirds of the cases there was no change in the prescription. The prescriptions were reversed (canceled) between 20% and 46% of the time. The

Table 4
Drug–drug interactions with high likelihood of clinical importance

Object drug or drug class	Precipitant drug or drug class	Interaction	Total number of cases among 46 million patients	Number of cases per 1000 exposed PBM plan participants: Object drug/precipitant drug
Anticoagulants (anisindione, dicumarol, warfarin)	Thyroid hormones	Increased risk of bleeding because of increased metabolism of vitamin K–dependent clotting factors. No increased risk if warfarin is started after patient is on stable thyroid hormone therapy	69,002	131.1/42.7
Benzodiazepines (alprazolam, triazolam)	Azole antifungals (fluconazole, itraconazole, ketoconazole)	Increased benzodiazepine concentration because of inhibition of CYP3A	91,567	44.5/70.1
Carbamazepine	Propoxyphene	Increased carbamazepine concentration because of decreased hepatic metabolism	9951	75/5
Cyclosporine	Rifamycins (rifampin, rifabutin, rifapentine)	Decreased CSA concentration because of induction of CYP enzymes	44	2.3/2.1
Dextromethorphan	MAO inhibitors (isocarboxazid, phenelzine, selegiline, tranylcypromine)	Increased risk of serotonin syndrome because of altered catecholamine uptake and metabolism	64	0.1/4.3
Digoxin	Clarithromycin	Increased digoxin concentration because of inhibition of p-glycoprotein	15,403	32.8/10.1
Ergot alkaloids	Macrolides (clarithromycin, erythromycin, troleandomycin) NOT azithromycin	Increased concentration of ergots because of inhibition of CYP3A	1679	71.5/0.6

Oral contraceptives	Rifampin	Decreased concentration of estrogens and progestin because of induction of CYP enzymes	559	0.2/26.9
Ganciclovir	Zidovudine	Increased risk of hematologic toxicities by unknown mechanism	102	28.7/4.8
Hydantoins	Dopamine	Risk for hypotension and MI is increased		Not in study
MAO inhibitors	Anorexiants	Increased risk for serotonin syndrome and hypertensive crisis because of increased norepinephrine availability	473	31.7/0.8
MAO inhibitors	Sympathomimetics	Increased risk for hypertensive crisis because of increased norepinephrine availability	427	28.7/0.1
Meperidine	MAO inhibitors	Increased risk for cardiovascular instability, hyperpyrexia, agitation, seizures, diaphoresis due to unknown mechanism	52	0.2/3.5
Metformin	Iodinated contrast agents	Increased risk for severe lactic acidosis		Not in study
Methotrexate	Trimethoprim	Increased risk for hematologic toxicity because of synergistic effect on folate metabolism	5044	56.2/2.4
Nitrates	Sildenafil, tadalafil, vardenafil	Increased hypotensive effect because of increased levels of cGMP	4811	5.9/17.9
Nondepolarizing muscle relaxants	Aminoglycosides	Prolonged neuromuscular blockade		Not in study
Pimozide	Macrolides	Increased risk for cardiotoxicity because of inhibition of CYP3A	90	44.3/0.03

(continued on next page)

Table 4 (*continued*)

Object drug or drug class	Precipitant drug or drug class	Interaction	Total number of cases among 46 million patients	Number of cases per 1000 exposed PBM plan participants Object drug/precipitant drug
Pimozide	Azole antifungals	Increased risk for cardiotoxicity because of inhibition of CYP3A	37	18.2/0.03
SSRIs	MAO inhibitors	Increased risk for serotonin syndrome because of inhibition of reuptake	1942	0.6/130.3
Theophylline	Fluoroquinolones (ciprofloxacin, enoxacin)	Increased concentration of theophylline because of inhibition of CYP1A2	50,284	224.5/13.8
Theophylline	Fluvoxamine	Increased concentration of theophylline because of inhibition of CYP1A2	152	0.7/4
Theophylline	Halothane	Theophylline concentration is increased because of inhibition of CYP2E1		Not in study
Thiopurines (azathioprine, mercaptopurine)	Allopurinol	Increased risk for thiopurine toxicity because of inhibition of xanthine oxidase	558	12.9/2.2

Warfarin	Sulfinpyrazone	Increased warfarin concentration and risk for bleeding because of impaired metabolism. Both are 2C9 substrates.	40	0.08/84.2
Warfarin	NSAIDs	Increased risk for bleeding because of gastric erosion and inhibition of platelet aggregation	127,684	242.7/15.9
Warfarin	Cimetidine	Increased warfarin concentration and risk for bleeding because of inhibition of CYP2C9	5547	10.6/19.5
Warfarin	Fibric acid derivatives (clofibrate, fenofibrate, gemfibrozil)	Increased risk for bleeding because of unknown mechanism	17,160	32.7/47.2
Warfarin	Barbiturates	Decreased warfarin concentration because of increased metabolism by CYP2C9	5172	9.9/27.7

Abbreviations: cGMP, cyclic guanosine monophasphate; CSA, cyclosporine A; MAO, monamine oxidase; MI, myocardial infarction; SMZ, sulfamethoxazole; SSRI, selective serotonin reuptake inhibitor; TMP, trimethoprim; TPN, parenteral nutrition.
Data from Refs. [45,48,62–64].

interaction of warfarin with NSAIDs was the most common and occurred in 127,684 cases. This represents an exposure of 242.7 patients per 1000 patients taking warfarin and 15.9 patients per 1000 patients taking NSAIDs (Table 4) [45,48,62–64]. Most potential interactions occurred in patients who were older than 50 years of age, and the exposure rate increased with increasing age.

Commonly prescribed drugs in critically ill patients

What constitutes commonly used drugs in critically ill patients vary by nation, region, type of hospital, and even by individual ICUs within a hospital [65]. Table 5 lists the 40 most commonly used drugs at the University of Minnesota-Fairview Medical Center in the surgical (SICU), medical (MICU) and pediatric (PICU) ICUs during the first quarter of 2005. There are 23 drugs among the top 40 used in the MICU that are not in the top 40 of the PICU and 13 that are not in the top 40 of the SICU. There are 8 drugs in the SICU top 40 that are not in the top 40 of the MICU or PICU. Over time the drugs that are used commonly in an ICU also change. Of the top 30 drugs in the author's ICUs in 1990, only 12 in the SICU, 12 in the MICU, and 14 in the PICU are still in the top 40 for those units today [2]. Variability is expected to increase in open admission ICUs, compared with closed ICUs. Common interacting drugs included macrolide antibiotics (not azithromycin), benzodiazepines (not lorazepam), HIV protease inhibitors, calcium channel blockers, and HMG CoA reductase inhibitors (not pravastatin), which are substrates for CYP3A4 and CYP3A5. β-Blockers, antidepressants, and antipsychotics are frequent substrates for CYP2D6. NSAIDs, oral hypoglycemics, and angiotensin II blockers (not candesartan or valsartan) are substrates for CYP2C9. The proton pump inhibitors and antiepileptics are primarily substrates for CYP2C19 [44].

Drug interaction management

The most common approach to minor drug interactions is to avoid the combination if possible, adjust the dose of the object drug, alter the administration times of the drugs to minimize the overlap, and closely monitor for early detection [66]. Another important step is to maintain current knowledge with respect to drug labeling. A study of trends in drug interactions for pharmaceutical products in Japan from January 2000 to December 2003 revealed a striking number of package insert changes were due to new information regarding drug interactions [67]. Of the 476 new drug interactions revisions that were reported, many (45%) were explanations of metabolic pathways and identification of CYP isoforms that are involved in the metabolic process. CYP3A4 was the primary isozyme involved (48% of revised package inserts), followed by CYP1A2 (14%), CYP2D6 (8%), CYP2C19 (2%), and CYP2C9 (1%). The cytochrome P isoform was not identified in 25% of the label revisions for drug

Table 5
Top 40 dispensed medications in the University of Minnesota Medical Center-Fairview ICUs from January to March 2005

Rank	Medical ICU	Surgical ICU	Pediatric ICU
1	IV solutions	IV solutions	IV solutions
2	Potassium	Magnesium	Potassium
3	Pantoprazole	Potassium	Heparin
4	Magnesium	Insulin	Bumetanide
5	Insulin	Pantoprazole	Furosemide
6	Lorazepam	Metoprolol	Calcium
7	Calcium	Furosemide	Pantoprazole
8	Heparin	Heparin	Aminophylline
9	Vancomycin	Hydromorphone	Ranitidine
10	Metoprolol	Ranitidine	Lorazepam
11	Fentanyl	Propofol	Vancomycin
12	Piperacillin/tazobactam	Vancomycin	Midazolam
13	Furosemide	Piperacillin/tazobactam	Chlorothiazide
14	Propofol	Aspirin	Fentanyl
15	Acetaminophen	Fentanyl	Methadone
16	Epoprostenol	Albuterol	Hydrocortisone
17	Imipenem/cilastatin	Sodium bicarbonate	Spironolactone
18	Metronidazole	Amiodarone	Intralipid
19	Hydrocortisone	Mycophenolate	Cefotaxime
20	Ranitidine	Epoetin	TPN
21	Albuterol	Oxycodone	Captopril
22	Prednisone	Lorazepam	Acetaminophen
23	Diltiazem	Albumin	Cefazolin
24	Metoclopramide	Cefazolin	Piperacillin/tazobactam
25	Sodium bicarbonate	Docusate	Metoclopramide
26	Methylprednisone	Morphine	Epinephrine
27	Multivitamin	Calcium	Albumin
28	Hydromorphone	Hydralazine	Nafcillin
29	Acetylcysteine	Tacrolimus	Ursodiol
30	Voriconazole	Methylprednisone	Tobramycin
31	Ciprofloxacin	Levofloxacin	Dexamethasone
32	Epoetin	Fluconazole	Prazosin
33	Methadone	Valproic acid	Chloral hydrate
34	Aspirin	Hydrocortisone	Albuterol
35	Valproic acid	Lidocaine	Phytonadione
36	Dornase	Prednisone	Iron
37	Morphine	TPN	Ceftazidime
38	Meropenem	Imipenem/cilastatin	Magnesium
39	Levofloxacin	SMZ/TMP	Sildenafil
40	Baclofen	Ursodiol	Diphenhydramine

Abbreviations: IV, intravenous; SMZ, sulfamethoxazole; TMP, trimethoprim; TPN, parenteral nutrition.

interactions. Revisions identified drugs as substrates for metabolic enzymes (65%), inhibitors of metabolic pathways (30%), or inducers of enzymes (5%). In many cases (40%) the references for the revision were company reports; 37% of references were published journals or books; and 24% of revisions did not cite any publications. Disappointingly, the time from publication of the reference to the revision of the package insert was more than 5 years in 58% of the cases.

Drug interaction software in hospitals should be improved to assist the clinician in identifying important and likely drug interactions. Eight strategies toward this end have been identified [68].

- Computer systems should interact so information on patient drug use from multiple pharmacy systems can be accessed in real time.
- Warnings in systems should be individualized so patient factors that increase the risk for a drug interaction (renal failure, liver failure, age) can be integrated in the severity decision.
- Trivial drug interactions should be defined and eliminated.
- New findings should be included in the software promptly.
- Inappropriate class-specific warnings should be eliminated because not all drugs in a class may undergo the drug interaction (macrolide antibiotics, statins, selective serotonin reuptake inhibitors).
- Optional links to more information should be available directly on the computer or through an Internet link.
- Rational therapeutic alternatives should be presented.
- Serious drug interactions should be more difficult to override and at least require authorization by a clinician.

Summary

Drug interactions are a significant clinical problem throughout health care. Critically ill patients are more vulnerable to drug interactions, including serious outcomes that may result. Many drug interactions result from the CYP450 enzyme system. Understanding the metabolic pathway of a drug can enhance one's ability to predict a drug interaction. When drug interactions are predicted the clinician has several therapeutic options, including adjusting drug dosages, substituting equivalent drugs with different pathways of elimination, temporarily discontinuing the interacting medication, and monitoring the patient for the predicted interaction. References and drug interaction software are improving in their ability to guide rational decision making when drug interaction potentials exist. There is an increasing knowledge base being generated by industry and required by the government of the mechanisms of drug interactions, but recognition and management of drug interactions can be improved [66,68].

Acknowledgments

The assistance of Dr. John Pastor, Assistant Director of Pharmacy at the University of Minnesota Medical Center-Fairview in obtaining the information on drug usage in the ICUs is gratefully acknowledged.

References

[1] Available at: http://www.ncbi.nlm.nih.gov/entrez/query.fcgi. Accessed December 29, 2005.
[2] Borchardt-Phelps PK, Mann HJ. Drug interactions in the ICU. Perspectives in Critical Care 1990;3:108–33.
[3] McInnes GT, Brodie MJ. Drug interactions that matter. A critical reappraisal. Drugs 1988;36: 83–110.
[4] Knijff-Dutmer EA, Schut GA, van de Laar MA. Concomitant coumarin-NSAID therapy and risk for bleeding. Ann Pharmacother 2003;37:12–6.
[5] Liu BA, Juurlink DN. Drugs and the QT interval–caveat doctor. N Engl J Med 2004;351: 1053–6.
[6] Juurlink DN, Mamdani M, Kopp A, et al. Drug-drug interactions among elderly patients hospitalized for drug toxicity. JAMA 2003;289:1652–8.
[7] Ray WA, Murray KT, Meredith S, et al. Oral erythromycin and the risk of sudden death from cardiac causes. N Engl J Med 2004;351:1089–96.
[8] Knijff-Dutmer EAJ, Postma MJ, van der Palen J, et al. Incremental cost-effectiveness of cyclo-oxygenase 2-selective versus nonselective nonsteroidal anti-inflammatory drugs in a cohort of coumarin users: a pharmacoeconomic analysis linked to a case-control study. Clin Ther 2004; 26:1160–7.
[9] Lasser KE, Allen PD, Woolhandler SJ, et al. Timing of new black box warnings and withdrawals for prescription medications. JAMA 2002;287:2215–20.
[10] Dimasi JA, Hansen RW, Grabowski HG. The price of innovation: new estimates of drug development costs. J Health Econ 2003;22:151–85.
[11] Lin JH, Lu AY. Interindividual variability in inhibition and induction of cytochrome P450 enzymes. Annu Rev Pharmacol Toxicol 2001;41:535–67.
[12] Rodrigues AD, Lin JH. Screening of drug candidates for their drug–drug interaction potential. Curr Opin Chem Biol 2001;5:396–401.
[13] Lin JH. Sense and nonsense in the prediction of drug-drug interactions. Curr Drug Metab 2000;1:305–31.
[14] Davit B, Reynolds K, Yuan R, et al. FDA evaluations using in vitro metabolism to predict and interpret in vivo metabolic drug-drug interactions: impact on labeling. J Clin Pharmacol 1999; 39:899–910.
[15] Wienkers LC. Factors confounding the successful extrapolation of in vitro CYP3A inhibition information to the in vivo condition. Eur J Pharm Sci 2002;15:239–42.
[16] Wienkers LC, Heath TG. Predicting in vivo drug interactions from in vitro drug discovery data. Nat Rev Drug Discov 2005;4:825–33.
[17] Bjornsson TD, Callaghan JT, Einolf HJ, et al. The conduct of in vitro and in vivo drug-drug interaction studies: a PhRMA perspective. J Clin Pharmacol 2003;43:443–69.
[18] Obach RS, Walsky RL, Venkatakrishnan K, et al. The utility of in vitro cytochrome p450 inhibition data in the prediction of drug-drug interactions. J Pharmacol Exp Ther 2006;316:336–48.
[19] Guidance for Industry. Drug metabolism/drug interaction studies in the drug development process: studies in vitro. Available at http://www.fda.gov/cder/guidance/clin3.pdf. Accessed January 23, 2006.
[20] Guidance for Industry. In vivo drug metabolism/drug interaction studies- study design, data analysis, and recommendations for dosing and labeling. Available at: http://www.fda.gov/cder/guidance/2635fnl.pdf. Accessed January 23, 2006.
[21] Marroum PJ, Gobburu J. The product label—how pharmacokinetics and pharmacodynamics reach the prescriber. Clin Pharmacokinet 2002;41:161–9.
[22] Marroum PJ, Uppoor RS, Parmelee T, et al. In vivo drug-drug interaction studies—a survey of all new molecular entities approved from 1987 to 1997. Clin Pharmacol Ther 2000;68:280–5.
[23] Lewis DF. 57 varieties: the human cytochromes P450. Pharmacogenomics 2004;5:305–18.
[24] Riddick DS. Drug biotranformation. In: Kalant H, Roschlau W, editors. Principles of medical pharmacology. 6th edition. New York: Oxford University Press; 1998. p. 38–54.

[25] Markey SP. Pathways of drug metabolism. In: Atkinson AJ, Daniels CE, Dedrick RL, et al, editors. Principles of clinical pharmacology. 1st edition. London: Academic Press; 2001. p. 123–42.
[26] Danielson PB. The cytochrome P450 superfamily: biochemistry, evolution and drug metabolism in humans. Curr Drug Metab 2002;3:561–97.
[27] Shimada T, Yamazaki H, Mimura M, et al. Interindividual variations in human liver cytochrome P-450 enzymes involved in the oxidation of drugs, carcinogens and toxic chemicals: studies with liver microsomes of 30 Japanese and 30 Caucasians. J Pharmacol Exp Ther 1994;270: 414–23.
[28] McKinnon RA, Burgess WM, Hall PM, et al. Characterisation of CYP3A gene subfamily expression in human gastrointestinal tissues. Gut 1995;36:259–67.
[29] Waxman DJ. P450 gene induction by structurally diverse xenochemicals: central role of nuclear receptors CAR, PXR, and PPAR. Arch Biochem Biophys 1999;369:11–23.
[30] Shapiro LE, Shear NH. Drug interactions: proteins, pumps, and P-450s. J Am Acad Dermatol 2002;47:467–84.
[31] Sikka R, Magauran B, Ulrich A, et al. Bench to bedside: pharmacogenomics, adverse drug interactions, and the cytochrome P450 system. Acad Emerg Med 2005;12:1227–35.
[32] de Leon J, Armstrong SC, Cozza KL. Clinical guidelines for psychiatrists for the use of pharmacogenetic testing for CYP450 2D6 and CYP450 2C19. Psychosomatics 2006;47:75–85.
[33] Kim K, Johnson JA, Derendorf H. Differences in drug pharmacokinetics between East Asians and Caucasians and the role of genetic polymorphisms. J Clin Pharmacol 2004;44: 1083–105.
[34] Cascorbi I. Pharmacogenetics of cytochrome p4502D6: genetic background and clinical implication. Eur J Clin Invest 2003;33(Suppl 2):17–22.
[35] Evans WE, McLeod HL. Pharmacogenomics—drug disposition, drug targets, and side effects. N Engl J Med 2003;348:538–49.
[36] Wilkinson GR. Drug metabolism and variability among patients in drug response. N Engl J Med 2005;352:2211–21.
[37] Lewis DF. Human cytochromes P450 associated with the phase 1 metabolism of drugs and other xenobiotics: a compilation of substrates and inhibitors of the CYP1, CYP2 and CYP3 families. Curr Med Chem 2003;10:1955–72.
[38] Elbekai RH, Korashy HM, El-Kadi AO. The effect of liver cirrhosis on the regulation and expression of drug metabolizing enzymes. Curr Drug Metab 2004;5:157–67.
[39] Korashy HM, Elbekai RH, El-Kadi AO. Effects of renal diseases on the regulation and expression of renal and hepatic drug-metabolizing enzymes: a review. Xenobiotica 2004;34:1–29.
[40] Villeneuve JP, Pichette V. Cytochrome P450 and liver diseases. Curr Drug Metab 2004;5: 273–82.
[41] Bastien MC, Leblond F, Pichette V, et al. Differential alteration of cytochrome P450 isoenzymes in two experimental models of cirrhosis. Can J Physiol Pharmacol 2000;78:912–9.
[42] Renton KW. Cytochrome P450 regulation and drug biotransformation during inflammation and infection. Curr Drug Metab 2004;5:235–43.
[43] Zhou S, Yung CS, Cher GB, et al. Mechanism-based inhibition of cytochrome P450 3A4 by therapeutic drugs. Clin Pharmacokinet 2005;44:279–304.
[44] Cytochrome P. 450 drug-interaction table. Available at: http://medicine.iupui.edu/flockhart/. Accessed January 24, 2006.
[45] Levien TL, Baker DE. Selected interactions caused by cytochrome P450 enzymes. Available at: http://www.pharmacistsletter.com. Accessed December 20, 2005.
[46] Package insert for Vaprisol (conivaptan hydrochloride injection). Available at: http://www.fda.gov/cder/foi/label/2005/021697lbl.pdf. Accessed January 27, 2006.
[47] Johnson MD, Newkirk G, White Jr JR. Clinically significant drug interactions. Postgrad Med 1999;105:193–6.
[48] Michalets EL. Update: clinically significant cytochrome P-450 drug interactions. Pharmacotherapy 1998;18:84–112.

[49] Mignat C. Clinically significant drug interactions with new immunosuppressive agents. Drug Saf 1997;16:267–78.
[50] Tanaka E. Clinically significant pharmacokinetic drug interactions between antiepileptic drugs. J Clin Pharm Ther 1999;24:87–92.
[51] Tanaka E, Hisawa S. Clinically significant pharmacokinetic drug interactions with psychoactive drugs: antidepressants and antipsychotics and the cytochrome P450 system. J Clin Pharm Ther 1999;24:7–16.
[52] Bentue-Ferrer D, Tribut O, Polard E, et al. Clinically significant drug interactions with cholinesterase inhibitors: a guide for neurologists. CNS Drugs 2003;17:947–63.
[53] Finch CK, Chrisman CR, Baciewicz AM, et al. Rifampin and rifabutin drug interactions: an update. Arch Intern Med 2002;162:985–92.
[54] Murphy JE, Forrey RA, DeSiraju U. Community pharmacists' responses to drug-drug interaction alerts. Am J Health Syst Pharm 2004;61:1484–7.
[55] Glintborg B, Andersen SE, Dalhoff K. Drug-drug interactions among recently hospitalised patients—frequent but mostly clinically insignificant. Eur J Clin Pharmacol 2005;61:675–81.
[56] Hansten PD, Horn JD. Drug interactions. Analysis and management. A clinical perspective and analysis of current developments. Facts and comparisons. St. Louis (MO): Wolters Kluwer Health; 2004.
[57] Doucet J, Chassagne P, Trivalle C, et al. Drug-drug interactions related to hospital admissions in older adults: a prospective study of 1000 patients. J Am Geriatr Soc 1996;44:944–8.
[58] Egger SS, Drewe J, Schlienger RG. Potential drug-drug interactions in the medication of medical patients at hospital discharge. Eur J Clin Pharmacol 2003;58:773–8.
[59] Jankel CA, Speedie SM. Detecting drug interactions: a review of the literature. DICP 1990;24: 982–9.
[60] Malone DC, Abarca J, Hansten PD, et al. Identification of serious drug-drug interactions: results of the partnership to prevent drug-drug interactions. J Am Pharm Assoc (Wash) 2004;44: 142–51.
[61] Abarca J, Malone DC, Armstrong EP, et al. Concordance of severity ratings provided in four drug interaction compendia. J Am Pharm Assoc (Wash) 2004;44:136–41.
[62] Malone DC, Hutchins DS, Haupert H, et al. Assessment of potential drug-drug interactions with a prescription claims database. Am J Health Syst Pharm 2005;62:1983–91.
[63] Drug Digest. Available at: http://www.drugdigest.org/DD/Home. Accessed December 12, 2005.
[64] Lesher BA. Clinically important drug interactions encountered in ambulatory and community pharmacy practices. Available at: http://www.pharmacistsletter.com. Accessed December 20, 2005.
[65] Mann HJ, Wittbrodt ET. Identifying drug usage patterns in the intensive care unit. Pharmacoeconomics 1993;4:235–9.
[66] Hansten PD. Drug interaction management. Pharm World Sci 2003;25:94–7.
[67] Yoshida N, Yamada A, Mimura Y, et al. Trends in new drug interactions for pharmaceutical products in Japan. Pharmacoepidemiol Drug Saf, in press.
[68] Juurlink DN. Drug-drug interactions: where do we go from here? J Am Pharm Assoc (Wash DC) 2004;44:128,131–2,134.

ELSEVIER
SAUNDERS

Crit Care Clin 22 (2006) 347–355

CRITICAL
CARE
CLINICS

Drug-Associated Disease: Hematologic Dysfunction

Erik R. Vandendries, MD, PhD[a,c,*], Reed E. Drews, MD[b,*]

[a]*Division of Hemostasis/Thrombosis, Beth Israel Deaconess Medical Center, Harvard Medical School, 330 Brookline Avenue, Boston, MA 02215, USA*
[b]*Division of Hematology-Oncology, Beth Israel Deaconess Medical Center, Harvard Medical School, 330 Brookline Avenue, Boston, MA 02215, USA*
[c]*PAREXEL International, 200 West Street, Waltham, MA 02451, USA*

Drug-induced hematologic dysfunction frequently complicates medical therapy. The severity of dysfunction can range from mild thrombocytopenia to aplastic anemia or catastrophic thrombosis. Initial management always involves stopping the offending drug, and other interventions are dictated by the specific hematologic complication. The most common drug-induced hematologic complications are cytopenias, including anemia, neutropenia, and thrombocytopenia. These cytopenias can be separated into two broad categories: those that result from decreased production in the bone marrow, and those that are caused by increased cell destruction (eg, drug-associated immune-mediated cytopenias). Other complications include hemorrhage, usually from severe thrombocytopenia or anticoagulants, and thrombosis, as in heparin-induced thrombocytopenia or drug-induced thrombotic microangiopathy.

Bone marrow underproduction cytopenias

A variety of drugs that is used in treating disease can affect hematopoiesis negatively and result in (1) pancytopenia, if the effect is at the level of the pluripotential hematopoietic stem cell; or (2) isolated cytopenias (anemia, neutro-

* Corresponding authors. PAREXEL International, 200 West Street, Waltham, MA 02451.
E-mail addresses: rdrews@bidmc.harvard.edu (R.E. Drews), Erik.Vandendries@parexel.com (E.R. Vandendries).

doi:10.1016/j.ccc.2006.02.002 ***criticalcare.theclinics.com***

penia or thrombocytopenia), if the problem involves a specific hematopoietic cell lineage (red blood cells [RBCs], granulocytes, or platelets). Certain drugs generally cause transient hematologic side effects, such as cytotoxic chemotherapies that are administered for malignancies. With other drugs, hematologic abnormalities may develop unexpectedly because of dose-independent mechanisms that are idiosyncratic and persist despite the discontinuation of the drug.

Aplastic anemia

Aplastic anemia is often idiopathic, but excluding drugs as the cause always poses a challenge [1,2]. With bone marrow injury, neutropenia occurs quickly with increased risk for infection (blood neutrophil survival is 7–10 hours); thrombocytopenia follows within days with mucocutaneous findings (petechiae, ecchymoses) and menometrorrhagia as manifestations of increased bleeding risk (platelet survival is 7–10 days); and anemia progresses slowly over weeks unless hastened by bleeding or hemolysis (RBC survival is 100–120 days). Drugs that are associated commonly with bone marrow aplasia include chloramphenicol, gold, nonsteroidal anti-inflammatory drugs (eg, phenylbutazone, indomethacin), sulfonamides, antiepileptic agents (eg, felbamate), and arsenicals [1]. When patients take numerous drugs it is difficult to identify the most likely drug that is responsible for the patient's bone marrow aplasia. In some instances, aplasia correlates with the total cumulative dose of drug administered as with gold [3].

Drug-induced aplasia arises by direct toxic effects of a drug on bone marrow or dose-independent idiosyncratic reactions to a drug [2]. When bone marrow aplasia relates to direct drug-induced myelotoxic effects, discontinuing the offending drug may resolve aplasia, whereas aplasia that is due to drug-induced idiosyncratic reactions generally is irreversible. Bone marrow aspiration and biopsy findings may suggest myelotoxic drug effects. For example, chloramphenicol can induce myelotoxic and idiosyncratic bone marrow suppression syndromes [4]. With a myelotoxic mechanism, vacuolated pronormoblasts appear, and the effects reverse upon discontinuation of the drug. Reduced multidrug resistance P-glycoprotein function may contribute to development of aplasia in some patients [5]; however, drug-induced aplasias that are related to idiosyncratic reactions are believed to be immune-mediated, with destruction of myeloid progenitors by lymphocytes [2]. In these instances, immunosuppressive therapies (eg, cyclosporine, antithymocyte globulin) may be beneficial [2]. Younger patients who have severe cytopenias and histocompatible donors may require hematopoietic stem-cell transplantation [2].

Myelodysplasia

Myelodysplasia, which transforms over time to acute myelogenous leukemia, may occur with certain drugs, such as high-dose or long-term alkylator use (eg, cyclophosphamide, chlorambucil) or topoisomerase II inhibitors (eg, etoposide, teniposide) [6,7]. Macrocytosis from idiopathic megaloblastic erythroid maturation suggests the development of a drug-induced myelodysplastic syndrome

(MDS). MDS usually produces bone marrow hypercellularity, but some patients have hypoplastic myelodysplasia, which is distinguished from aplastic anemia by bone marrow cytogenetics [2].

Macrocytosis also may arise from inhibition of DNA synthesis by certain drugs, which acts by inhibiting intestinal absorption of folate or cobalamin or by inhibiting enzymes that are required in folate metabolism or DNA synthesis. For example, neomycin, biguanides (eg, metformin), and proton pump inhibitors (eg, omeprazole) block intestinal absorption of cobalamin. Phenytoin, methotrexate, and trimethoprim inhibit folate metabolism. Certain drugs alter nucleotide pools, which results in slowed DNA synthesis and delayed nuclear maturation in relation to cytoplasmic maturation, the hallmark of megaloblastosis. Such drugs include hydroxyurea (which inhibits ribonucleotide reductase), methotrexate (which inhibits dihydrofolate reductase), zidovudine, azathioprine (a prodrug of 6-mercaptopurine), other purine nucleoside analogs (eg, fludarabine, cladribine), and other antineoplastic agents.

Enzyme deficiencies and drug-induced myelosuppression

With azathioprine or 6-mercaptopurine use, 0.3% of patients develop macrocytosis and severe bone marrow suppression that are due to inherited homozygous deficiency of thiopurine methyltransferase (TPMT), an enzyme that is required in azathioprine metabolism [8]. Heterozygous deficiency of TPMT is seen in 11% of patients; these individuals also have increased risks for azathioprine or 6-mercaptopurine-induced myelosuppression [8]. With 5-fluorouracil use, 3% to 5% of whites and 0.1% of African Americans develop severe pancytopenia (as well as mucositis, diarrhea, and neurotoxicity) because of an inherited deficiency of dihydropyrimidine dehydrogenase, an enzyme that is required in pyrimidine metabolism [9,10]. Certain patients may require genotypic and phenotypic assessments of these enzyme deficiencies [8,11].

Drug-induced erythropoietin deficiency

Cisplatin therapy results chiefly in anemia, with lesser effects on neutrophils and platelets. This hematologic effect correlates with reduced serum erythropoietin (EPO) levels following cisplatin use, which are lower than expected for the observed degree of anemia [12]. Reduced EPO production during cisplatin therapy arises from reversible cisplatin-induced renal tubular damage, and endogenous EPO production recovers with discontinuation of cisplatin therapy [12].

Recombinant EPO (rEPO) rarely induces neutralizing antibodies, which eliminate endogenous EPO and exogenous rEPO response, and result in pure red cell aplasia (PRCA) [13,14]. Most patients have had chronic renal failure and received subcutaneous administration of rEPO [13]. Hematologic findings include hemoglobin levels declining by 0.7 to 1 mg/dL per week, reticulocytopenia (absolute reticulocyte counts $<10{,}000/\mu L$), and absent to near absent erythroid progenitors on bone marrow biopsy. Incident rates of rEPO-associated PRCA are10-fold greater in patients who receive Eprex, a human serum albumin-free formulation of epoetin α that is manufactured and distributed outside of the United States [13]. Incident rates are far lower with the epoetin β formulation NeoRecormon (stabilized with polysorbate 20) and the epoetin α formulation Epogen (Procrit) [13]. In the case of Eprex, immunogenicity to rEPO may relate to organic compounds leached from uncoated rubber stoppers in prefilled syringes that contained polysorbate 80 [15]. With use of Teflon-coated stoppers and administration of Eprex intravenously (rather than subcutaneously), the exposure-adjusted incidence rates of PRCA that are due to Eprex have decreased 13-fold [13]. The basis for neutralizing antibody development in patients who receive Epogen or Procrit is unknown.

Drug-induced immune cytopenias

Drug-induced cytopenias, including thrombocytopenia, neutropenia, and anemia, often are associated with an immune-related increase in blood cell destruction. The mechanism of immune-related destruction of blood cells varies and can involve direct antidrug antibodies, antibodies that are directed against the drug complexed with other protein(s), or antibodies against a component of the blood cell independent of drug. For example, in penicillin-induced hemolytic anemia, the penicillins bind plasma and RBC membrane proteins to form a complex in which the penicillin molecule acts as a hapten in an immune response. Antibodies that are directed against the penicillin can induce hemolytic anemia by binding to the penicillin that is bound to the RBC membrane. Usually, in penicillin-induced hemolytic anemia, the direct antiglobulin test is positive, whereas the indirect antiglobulin test is negative. Other drugs, such as methyldopa and procainamide, induce antibodies that bind RBC membrane antigens and cause autoimmune hemolytic anemia independent of immune complex formation with drug or drug metabolite [16].

Penicillin-induced thrombocytopenia also occurs. As another example of drug-induced thrombocytopenia, quinine seems to produce a conformational change on platelet-specific antigens (glycoprotein (GP)IIb/IIIa and GPIb/IX), which then become immunogenic [17]. The quinine-induced antiplatelet antibodies can cause severe thrombocytopenia, often 5 to 8 days after exposure to quinine. Quinine-induced hemolytic anemia, neutropenia, and thrombotic thrombocytopenia purpura (TTP) also have been reported [16]. Drugs that are targeted to the GPIIb/IIIa complex, such as tirofiban and eptifibatide, can cause preexisting antibodies to bind to the GPIIb/IIIa complex, which produces acute thrombocytopenia.

Compared with drug-induced immune hemolytic anemia and thrombocytopenia, drug-induced immune neutropenia is rare. Nevertheless, such drugs as antithyroid medications (eg, propylthiouracil), clozapine, ticlopidine, sulfasalazine, and trimethoprim-sulfamethoxazole pose the highest risks for developing neutropenia. Antineutrophil antibodies in these instances depend on the drug or drug metabolite as hapten [18–20].

Heparin-induced thrombocytopenia

Heparin is an anticoagulant that is used frequently to prevent and treat thromboembolic disease, particularly in the critical care setting. Heparin acts by binding to antithrombin III. The resulting complex binds to and inhibits thrombin and factors IXa, Xa, and XIa [21]. Bleeding can complicate heparin anticoagulation, an effect that protamine can reverse. Heparin often causes asymptomatic mild thrombocytopenia. It also can induce more severe thrombocytopenia (heparin-induced thrombocytopenia [HIT]), which is mediated by heparin-induced antibodies that are directed against platelet factor 4–heparin complexes (PF4) and heightens the risk for thrombosis. The macromolecular complex of immunoglobulin, PF4, and heparin binds to and activates platelets, which subsequently release additional platelet agonists and procoagulant microparticles. These activated platelets and procoagulant microparticles are hypothesized to result in venous and arterial thrombosis. The risk of HIT is highest with unfractionated heparin in the postoperative setting; pregnancy is associated with a lower risk. In contrast to unfractionated heparin, low molecular weight heparin (LMWH) is associated with a much lower risk for HIT development; however, LMWH cross-reacts with HIT antibodies that develop on exposure to unfractionated heparin, and the use of LMWH in this setting is contraindicated.

Diagnosing HIT requires correlating certain clinical features with laboratory findings. Thrombocytopenia, defined as a 50% or greater decline from baseline platelet counts, is the most common finding. Typically, the severity of thrombocytopenia in HIT is moderate, with platelet counts around 50,000/mL [22]. In most patients without a recent previous exposure to heparin, the platelet count decreases approximately 5 to 10 days after exposure. In patients with a recent heparin exposure, the platelet count can decrease immediately. In another minority of patients, delayed onset-thrombocytopenia can occur days after the discontinuation of heparin [22,23]. Because heparin use and thrombocytopenia often occur in patients who take multiple medications, clinicians should consider other causes—particularly when thrombocytopenia is severe—because severe thrombocytopenia in HIT is unusual.

As a consequence of the antibody-mediated platelet activation, thrombosis is a frequent and worrisome finding in HIT. Most thrombotic events are venous thromboses; however, arterial thrombotic events do occur, including stroke and myocardial infarction. Other less common clinical findings include skin lesions at the sites of subcutaneous injections of heparin, warfarin-induced gangrene, and acute systemic reactions.

Laboratory findings include thrombocytopenia as described above. Fragmented RBCs and other indications of disseminated intravascular coagulation (DIC) usually are not seen. In addition to the above clinical findings, the diagnosis of HIT usually requires confirmation with an anti-PF4/heparin antibody immunoassay or a serotonin release assay [24]. The immunoassay is performed more frequently because it is less labor intensive and is available more readily. In this assay, the patient's serum is incubated with PF4/heparin complexes that are bound to microtiter plates. The amount of bound HIT antibody is detected and quantitated using an enzyme-linked anti-IgG antibody. Its specificity and sensitivity depend on the cutoff that is used to separate positive results from negative results. In the serotonin release assay, the patient's serum is incubated with heparin and washed platelets that contain radiolabeled serotonin. The amount of released serotonin determines a positive test. Although the serotonin release assay generally is considered to have a higher specificity (~98%) than the immunoassay (specificity of ~80%), it is more technically difficult and less available [25].

When HIT is confirmed or suspected, patients should discontinue all sources of heparin. Risk for thrombosis from HIT is high. Therefore, patients should receive an alternative anticoagulant to treat thrombosis that arises from HIT or to prevent thrombosis after HIT is diagnosed. US Food and Drug Administration–approved anticoagulants that are used for treating HIT include lepirudin and argatroban [24]. Lepirudin and argatroban are direct thrombin inhibitors and prolong the activated partial thromboplastin time (aPTT), but they have different pharmacokinetics. Lepirudin should be used cautiously in patients who have renal failure, and argatroban is potentially problematic in patients who have liver dysfunction. Bivalirudin, another direct thrombin inhibitor, also can treat HIT. Fondaparinux, a synthetic pentasaccharide that inhibits factor Xa in an antithrombin III–dependent manner and does not seem to interact in a deleterious way with HIT antibodies, has been used in patients who have HIT [26]; however, limited data exist on its use and safety. Patients only should receive warfarin anticoagulation after platelet counts have returned to normal on one of the above anticoagulants.

Drug-induced thrombotic thrombocytopenia purpura/hemolytic uremia syndrome

The thrombotic microangiopathies include TTP and hemolytic uremia syndrome (HUS). Both are characterized by thrombocytopenia and microangiopathic hemolytic anemia with formation of platelet-rich microthrombi in the microvasculature [27]. Clinical manifestations of TTP usually include fever and neurologic manifestations (eg, headaches, somnolence, confusion, seizures). Typically, HUS is associated with renal dysfunction, without fever and neurologic symptoms or signs. Laboratory abnormalities include thrombocytopenia, elevated lactate dehydrogenase levels, and numerous fragmented RBCs (so-called "schistocytes") on peripheral blood smear. Elevations of the prothrombin time and aPTT are not expected because these findings suggest a consumptive coagulopathy, as in DIC. Although TTP and HUS may be idiopathic, familial, or induced by infections or malignancies, multiple drugs are associated with both conditions [28,29]. Implicated drugs include clopidogrel, ticlopidine, cyclosporine, and certain chemotherapeutic agents, such as gemcitabine, mitomycin-C, and cisplatin.

The antiplatelet agents clopidogrel and ticlopidine are associated with the development of TTP [30,31]. Initially, ticlopidine was linked with TTP in 1991 and is now believed to have occurred in at least 1 in 5000 patients who used ticlopidine. Clopidogrel, a newer ADP receptor antagonist, also seems to be associated with TTP, albeit with a lower incidence. Clopidogrel- and ticlopidine-induced TTP can occur with an immune-mediated decrease in a disintegrin and metalloprotinase with thrombospondin motifs-13 activity [30,32]. The preferred treatment remains plasma exchange with a mortality of 9% to 18% [30].

Although malignancy can cause TTP or HUS, certain chemotherapeutic agents may have an independent association with TTP or HUS. Mitomycin-C–associated TTP is characterized by microangiopathic hemolytic anemia, thrombocytopenia, renal failure, and dyspnea [33]. It can occur weeks after discontinuation of the drug and appears more frequently after cumulative doses of mitomycin-C. It has a particularly poor prognosis, and usually does not respond to plasma exchange. Multiple case reports implicate other chemotherapeutic drugs, including gemcitabine and cisplatin, in the development of HUS [34–36]. Quinine, a common cause of thrombocytopenia, can precipitate TTP [28,33]; quinine may induce antibody formation against GPIIb/IIIa and GPIb/IX and against endothelial and white blood cell antigens. Patients who have quinine-induced TTP have had microangiopathic hemolytic anemia, thrombocytopenia, fever, renal dysfunction, and neurologic abnormalities. TTP can occur quickly (within hours) after exposure to quinine. Treatment includes cessation of the drug and plasma exchange.

Anticoagulants

A major complication of anticoagulation is bleeding. The risk for major bleeding from warfarin, targeted to an international normalized ratio [INR] of 2.0 to 3.0, is approximately 1% per year. This risk of bleeding increases with age, aspirin use (and possibly with the use of other antiplatelet agents), hypertension, cerebral vascular disease, and malignancy [37]. An increasing INR, particularly greater than 4.0, exacerbates the risk for hemorrhage. Vitamin K can reverse warfarin anticoagulation; however, fresh frozen plasma should be used for the rapid reversal of warfarin-induced anticoagulation that is associated with life-threatening bleeding complications. Similarly, LMWH, and newer anticoagulants, such as fondaparinux, can heighten the risk for major bleeding [37]. Protamine can reverse heparin-induced anticoagulation, but protamine only partially reverses LMWH-induced anticoagulation, and does not reverse other anticoagulants, such as fondaparinux [38]. Preliminary evidence suggests that recombinant factor VIIa can reverse warfarin-induced anticoagulation and possibly LWMH or fondaparinux-induced anticoagulation [39,40].

References

[1] Kaufman DW, Kelly JP, Jurgelon JM, et al. Drugs in the aetiology of agranulocytosis and aplastic anaemia. Eur J Haematol Suppl 1996;60:23–30.

[2] Young NS. Acquired aplastic anemia. Ann Intern Med 2002;136(7):534–46.
[3] Kay AG. Myelotoxicity of gold. BMJ 1976;1(6020):1266–8.
[4] Wallerstein RO, Condit PK, Kasper CK, et al. Statewide study of chloramphenicol therapy and fatal aplastic anemia. JAMA 1969;208(11):2045–50.
[5] Calado RT, Garcia AB, Gallo DA, et al. Reduced function of the multidrug resistance P-glycoprotein in CD34+ cells of patients with aplastic anaemia. Br J Haematol 2002;118(1): 320–6.
[6] Pedersen-Bjergaard J. Radiotherapy- and chemotherapy-induced myelodysplasia and acute myeloid leukemia. A review. Leuk Res 1992;16(1):61–5.
[7] Sobecks RM, Le Beau MM, Anastasi J, et al. Myelodysplasia and acute leukemia following high-dose chemotherapy and autologous bone marrow or peripheral blood stem cell transplantation. Bone Marrow Transplant 1999;23(11):1161–5.
[8] Relling MV, Hancock ML, Rivera GK, et al. Mercaptopurine therapy intolerance and heterozygosity at the thiopurine S-methyltransferase gene locus. J Natl Cancer Inst 1999;91(23):2001–8.
[9] Harris BE, Carpenter JT, Diasio RB. Severe 5-fluorouracil toxicity secondary to dihydropyrimidine dehydrogenase deficiency. A potentially more common pharmacogenetic syndrome. Cancer 1991;68(3):499–501.
[10] Takimoto CH, Lu ZH, Zhang R, et al. Severe neurotoxicity following 5-fluorouracil-based chemotherapy in a patient with dihydropyrimidine dehydrogenase deficiency. Clin Cancer Res 1996;2(3):477–81.
[11] Ezzeldin H, Johnson MR, Okamoto Y, et al. Denaturing high performance liquid chromatography analysis of the DPYD gene in patients with lethal 5-fluorouracil toxicity. Clin Cancer Res 2003;9(8):3021–8.
[12] Wood PA, Hrushesky WJ. Cisplatin-associated anemia: an erythropoietin deficiency syndrome. J Clin Invest 1995;95(4):1650–9.
[13] Bennett CL, Cournoyer D, Carson KR, et al. Long-term outcome of individuals with pure red cell aplasia and antierythropoietin antibodies in patients treated with recombinant epoetin: a follow-up report from the Research on Adverse Drug Events and Reports (RADAR) Project. Blood 2005;106(10):3343–7.
[14] Bennett CL, Luminari S, Nissenson AR, et al. Pure red-cell aplasia and epoetin therapy. N Engl J Med 2004;351(14):1403–8.
[15] Boven K, Stryker S, Knight J, et al. The increased incidence of pure red cell aplasia with an Eprex formulation in uncoated rubber stopper syringes. Kidney Int 2005;67(6):2346–53.
[16] Aster RH. Drug-induced immune cytopenias. Toxicology 2005;209(2):149–53.
[17] Burgess JK. Molecular mechanisms of drug-induced thrombocytopenia. Curr Opin Hematol 2001;8(5):294–8.
[18] Berliner N, Horwitz M, Loughran Jr TP. Congenital and acquired neutropenia. Hematology (Am Soc Hematol Educ Program) 2004:63–79.
[19] Meyer O, Gaedicke G, Salama A. Demonstration of drug-dependent antibodies in two patients with neutropenia and successful treatment with granulocyte-colony-stimulating factor. Transfusion 1999;39(5):527–30.
[20] Salama A, Schutz B, Kiefel V, et al. Immune-mediated agranulocytosis related to drugs and their metabolites: mode of sensitization and heterogeneity of antibodies. Br J Haematol 1989;72(2): 127–32.
[21] Hirsh J, Raschke R, Warkentin TE, et al. Heparin: mechanism of action, pharmacokinetics, dosing considerations, monitoring, efficacy, and safety. Chest 1995;108(4 Suppl):258S–75S.
[22] Warkentin TE. New approaches to the diagnosis of heparin-induced thrombocytopenia. Chest 2005;127(2 Suppl):35S–45S.
[23] Warkentin TE, Bernstein RA. Delayed-onset heparin-induced thrombocytopenia and cerebral thrombosis after a single administration of unfractionated heparin. N Engl J Med 2003;348(11): 1067–9.
[24] Warkentin TE. Heparin-induced thrombocytopenia: diagnosis and management. Circulation 2004;110(18):e454–8.

[25] Menajovsky LB. Heparin-induced thrombocytopenia: clinical manifestations and management strategies. Am J Med 2005;118(Suppl 8A):21S–30S.
[26] Savi P, Chong BH, Greinacher A, et al. Effect of fondaparinux on platelet activation in the presence of heparin-dependent antibodies: a blinded comparative multicenter study with unfractionated heparin. Blood 2005;105(1):139–44.
[27] Moake JL. Thrombotic microangiopathies. N Engl J Med 2002;347(8):589–600.
[28] Dlott JS, Danielson CF, Blue-Hnidy DE, et al. Drug-induced thrombotic thrombocytopenic purpura/hemolytic uremic syndrome: a concise review. Ther Apher Dial 2004;8(2):102–11.
[29] McCarthy LJ, Dlott JS, Orazi A, et al. Thrombotic thrombocytopenic purpura: yesterday, today, tomorrow. Ther Apher Dial 2004;8(2):80–6.
[30] Bennett CL, Connors JM, Carwile JM, et al. Thrombotic thrombocytopenic purpura associated with clopidogrel. N Engl J Med 2000;342(24):1773–7.
[31] Bennett CL, Weinberg PD, Rozenberg-Ben-Dror K, et al. Thrombotic thrombocytopenic purpura associated with ticlopidine. A review of 60 cases. Ann Intern Med 1998;128(7):541–4.
[32] Tsai HM. Current concepts in thrombotic thrombocytopenic purpura. Annu Rev Med 2006;57:419–36.
[33] Medina PJ, Sipols JM, George JN. Drug-associated thrombotic thrombocytopenic purpura-hemolytic uremic syndrome. Curr Opin Hematol 2001;8(5):286–93.
[34] Jackson AM, Rose BD, Graff LG, et al. Thrombotic microangiopathy and renal failure associated with antineoplastic chemotherapy. Ann Intern Med 1984;101(1):41–4.
[35] Canpolat C, Pearson P, Jaffe N. Cisplatin-associated hemolytic uremic syndrome. Cancer 1994;74(11):3059–62.
[36] Fung MC, Storniolo AM, Nguyen B, et al. A review of hemolytic uremic syndrome in patients treated with gemcitabine therapy. Cancer 1999;85(9):2023–32.
[37] Levine MN, Raskob G, Beyth RJ, et al. Hemorrhagic complications of anticoagulant treatment: the Seventh ACCP Conference on Antithrombotic and Thrombolytic Therapy. Chest 2004;126(3 Suppl):287S–310S.
[38] Warkentin TE, Crowther MA. Reversing anticoagulants both old and new. Can J Anaesth 2002;49(6):S11–25.
[39] Hu Q, Brady JO. Recombinant activated factor VII for treatment of enoxaparin-induced bleeding. Mayo Clin Proc 2004;79(6):827.
[40] Freeman WD, Brott TG, Barrett KM, et al. Recombinant factor VIIa for rapid reversal of warfarin anticoagulation in acute intracranial hemorrhage. Mayo Clin Proc 2004;79(12):1495–500.

ELSEVIER
SAUNDERS

Crit Care Clin 22 (2006) 357–374

CRITICAL
CARE
CLINICS

Drug-Associated Renal Dysfunction

Stephanie S. Taber, PharmD*, Bruce A. Mueller, PharmD

Department of Clinical Sciences, University of Michigan College of Pharmacy, 1500 East Medical Center Drive, UHB2D301 Box 0008, Ann Arbor, MI 48109, USA

The development of acute renal failure (ARF) that requires renal replacement therapy is one of the most catastrophic events that can occur in a critically ill patient. ARF occurs in approximately 6% of patients in the ICU [1]. The mortality of patients in the ICU who require any type of renal replacement is greater than 50% [1]; this rate has not changed since the advent of dialysis [2]. Preexisting renal disease and left ventricular dysfunction have been identified as risk factors for the development of ARF [3]. Although clinicians recognize the seriousness of ARF in the ICU, little has been done to assess the overall contribution that pharmacotherapy has on the development of ARF. Sepsis generally is regarded as the most common cause of ARF in the ICU [4], but clinicians recognize that drug therapies are important contributors to renal dysfunction in the ICU. One small case series estimated that up to 14% of all cases of ARF in the ICU were caused by drugs [4]. It is difficult to determine the overall contribution of drug-induced renal dysfunction in the ICU because of the complexity of critically ill patients. Many of the essential drugs in the ICU (eg, antibiotics, vasopressors, intravenous contrast dye) are widely known to be nephrotoxic, yet they continue to be used because less toxic agents are unavailable or are less effective. To determine how often potentially nephrotoxic drugs are used in the ICUs in the authors' own institution, a brief drug use evaluation was conducted.

* Corresponding author.
E-mail address: staber@umich.edu (S.S. Taber).

doi:10.1016/j.ccc.2006.02.003 *criticalcare.theclinics.com*

Methods

The University of Michigan Health System (UMHS) is a tertiary care center with 865 licensed beds (550 adult, 206 pediatric). UMHS has 90 beds in six adult ICUs and 65 beds in three pediatric ICUs (Table 1), and is a Level 1 Trauma Center. Adult ICUs include medical intensive care, neurology intensive care, surgical intensive care, cardiac intensive care, thoracic surgery, and a trauma burn center. The pediatric ICUs consist of a neonatal ICU, pediatric ICU, and a cardiothoracic ICU. UMHS operates under a closed formulary system, and clinical pharmacists provide service to most of the ICU beds in the health system.

Through the pharmacy's order entry system the authors determined the top 100 drugs ordered, including scheduled and "as needed" medications, in each ICU during 2004. The lists from the adult ICUs were compiled into a master adult ICU drug list, and the lists from all of the pediatric ICUs were compiled into a master pediatric ICU drug list. If a drug was in the top 100 of any ICU, it appears in the master list. After these master lists were compiled, 182 different drugs appeared on the adult ICU master drug list and 151 drugs appeared on the pediatric ICU master drug list.

Each of the drugs on the list was evaluated for its nephrotoxic potential by the authors using the Micromedex drug information system [5]. Those drugs on the master list that had nephrotoxic potential were identified. Table 2 contains the nephrotoxic drugs that were in the top 100 used drugs in at least one of the adult ICUs. Table 3 contains the nephrotoxic drugs that were in the top 100 used drugs in at least one of the pediatric ICUs.

Results

Of the 182 different medications that were identified in any of the top 100 drug lists in the adult ICUs, 41 (22.5%) have nephrotoxic potential (see Table 2).

Table 1
University of Michigan adult and pediatric ICUs

ICU	# of beds
Adult	
Cardiac	10
Medical	20
Neurology	10
Surgical	20
Thoracic	14
Trauma/burn	16
Pediatric	
Cardiothoracic	12
Neonatal	37
Pediatric	16

Table 2
Most commonly prescribed medications in University of Michigan's adult ICUs

Drug name	# of times ordered	Primary mechanisms of nephrotoxicity
Acetaminophen	2751	AIN
Acetaminophen/codeine	262	AIN
Acetaminophen/hydrocodone	831	AIN
Acyclovir	99	ON
Allopurinol	34	Nephrolithiasis, AIN
Ampicillin/Sulbactam	411	AIN
Aspirin	1935	AIN, HD, NS
Azathioprine	28	AIN
Aztreonam	64	AIN
Bacitracin	390	ATN
Bacitracin/polymyxin	23	ATN
Captopril	170	AIN, HD
Carbamazepine	37	AIN
Cefazolin	1083	AIN
Cefepime	65	AIN
Cefotetan	94	AIN
Cefoxitin	159	AIN
Ceftazidime	36	AIN
Ceftriaxone	325	AIN
Ciprofloxacin	189	AIN
Cyclosporine	47	HD, CIN
Dopamine	512	HD
Epinephrine	62	HD
Furosemide	2085	AIN
Gentamicin	327	AIN, ATN
Hydrochlorothiazide	199	AIN
Ibuprofen	232	AIN, HD, NS, PN, MN
Ketorolac	181	AIN, HD, NS, PN, MN
Lisinopril	571	HD
Mannitol	67	Osmotic nephrosis, HD
Nafcillin	53	AIN
Omeprazole	384	AIN
Oxycodone/acetaminophen	29	AIN
Phenytoin	591	AIN
Piperacillin/tazobactam	1258	AIN
Rifampin	40	AIN
Sulfamethoxazole/trimethoprim	316	AIN, ON
Tacrolimus	86	HD, CIN
Topiramate	26	Nephrolithiasis
Vancomycin	1890	AIN
Warfarin	238	AIN, cholesterol emboli

Abbreviations: AIN, allergic interstitial nephritis; ATN, acute tubular necrosis; CIN, chronic interstitial necrosis; HD, hemodynamically mediated; MN, medullary necrosis; NS, nephrotic syndrome; ON, obstructive nephropathy; PN, papillary necrosis.

Table 3
Most commonly prescribed nephrotoxic medications in University of Michigan's pediatric ICUs

Drug name	# of times ordered	Primary mechanisms of nephrotoxicity
Acetaminophen	1083	AIN
Acetaminophen/codeine	139	AIN
Acyclovir	67	ON
Amoxicillin	56	AIN
Amphotericin B	17	ATN
Ampicillin	823	AIN
Ampicillin/sulbactam	411	AIN
Aspirin	1935	AIN, HD, NS
Bacitracin	124	ATN
Captopril	161	AIN, HD
Cefazolin	729	AIN
Cefotaxime	143	AIN
Cefotetan	9	AIN
Ceftazidime	14	AIN
Ceftriaxone	177	AIN
Cefuroxime	78	AIN
Chlorothiazide	408	AIN
Dopamine	753	HD
Enalapril	22	AIN, HD
Epinephrine	420	HD
Furosemide	960	AIN
Gentamicin	981	AIN, ATN
Ibuprofen	37	AIN, HD, NS, PN, MN
Immune globulin	5	Osmotic nephrosis
Indomethacin	35	AIN, HD, NS, PN, MN
Ketorolac	181	AIN, HD, NS, PN, MN
Levofloxacin	44	AIN
Mannitol	26	Osmotic nephrosis, HD
Omeprazole	61	AIN
Phenobarbital	282	AIN
Phenytoin	91	AIN
Piperacillin/tazobactam	174	AIN
Propanolol	12	HD
Rifampin	11	AIN
Sulfamethoxazole/trimethoprim	131	AIN, ON
Tacrolimus	57	HD, CIN
Vancomycin	477	AIN
Warfarin	19	AIN, cholesterol emboli

Abbreviations: AIN, allergic interstitial nephritis; ATN, acute tubular necrosis; CIN, chronic interstitial necrosis; HD, hemodynamically mediated; MN, medullary necrosis; NS, nephrotic syndrome; ON, obstructive nephropathy; PN, papillary necrosis.

The 182 drugs on the adult ICU master list accounted for 83,970 medication orders. The 41 potentially nephrotoxic drugs accounted for 21.6% of the total orders (18,180/83,970) in the adult ICUs. The pediatric master list contained 151 medications, of which 38 (25.2%) could cause kidney damage (see Table 3). In 2004, 27,924 medication orders that contained any of the 151 drugs on the pediatric master list were written in the pediatric ICUs. The nephrotoxic medication orders accounted for 39.9% (11,153/27,924) of the most commonly prescribed pediatric orders in the ICUs. The drugs that were used in the adult and pediatric ICUs differed substantially. Seventy-five of the 182 drugs that appeared in the top 100 in any of the adult ICUs did not appear in any of the pediatric ICU top 100 lists. Conversely, 46 of 151 top 100 pediatric ICU medications did not appear in any of the adult ICU top 100 lists. Similarly, 15 of the top 100 adult medications that were potential nephrotoxins that did not appear in the pediatric list, and 12 of the top 100 pediatric nephrotoxic medications did not appear in the adult list.

Discussion

The authors' brief evaluation of prescribing in the ICUs revealed that potentially nephrotoxic agents are used commonly in the adult and pediatric ICUs. The contrast media agents is one group of commonly nephrotoxic agents that the review was unable to quantify. In the authors' institution, contrast dye is not purchased or dispensed by the pharmacy; consequently the pharmacy tracking software did not capture its usage. Therefore, the use of potentially nephrotoxic agents is even higher than what is reported here.

The authors observed in the adult ICUs that the percentage of top 100 drugs prescribed that were potentially nephrotoxic (22.2%) was approximately the same as the number of actual orders written for these drugs (21.9%). In contrast, 25.2% of the drugs on the pediatric ICU list were potentially nephrotoxic, but these medications accounted for almost 40% of all medication orders in the pediatric ICUs. It is a commonly held clinical belief that children are less prone to nephrotoxicity; some studies suggested that drugs that are considered to be nephrotoxic in adults, are rarely nephrotoxic in children [6]. This concept of critically ill children having more "renal reserve" than critically ill adults may be true. Adults often have more comorbidities than do children. It is possible that pediatric intensivists are more comfortable in prescribing potential nephrotoxins than are their counterparts in the adult ICU. Less nephrotoxic alternatives may not be available for pediatric patients.

This medication use evaluation did not assess the nephrotoxicity rate of each prescribed agent; many of these identified potential nephrotoxins rarely cause drug-induced renal dysfunction. For example, acetaminophen-containing medications were considered to be potentially nephrotoxic; however, actual renal dysfunction from conventionally dosed acetaminophen is exceedingly rare. Nonetheless, the use of nephrotoxic agents, such as nonsteroidal anti-inflammatory drugs (NSAIDs), cephalosporins, penicillins, acyclovir, amphotericin B, aminoglycosides, and contrast dye are prevalent in the authors' ICUs. In this article, the respective methods of drug-induced renal dysfunction are described for these agents (Box 1).

Box 1. Medications that cause drug-induced renal dysfunction and sites of toxicity in critically ill patients

Hemodynamically mediated

- Angiotensin-converting enzyme inhibitors
- Angiotensin II receptor blockers
- NSAIDs

Glomerular disease

- Nephrotic syndrome
  - NSAIDs
- Glomerulonephritis
  - Hydralazine

Tubular epithelial cell damage

- Acute tubular necrosis
  - Aminoglycosides
  - Amphotericin B
  - Cisplatin/carboplatin
  - Radiographic contrast media
- Osmotic nephrosis
  - Immune globulin
  - Mannitol

Tubulointerstitial disease

- Acute allergic interstitial nephritis
  - See Box 2
- Chronic interstitial nephritis
  - Cyclosporine
- Papillary necrosis
  - NSAIDs

Obstructive nephropathy

- Intratubular obstruction
  - Acyclovir
  - Foscarnet
  - Indinavir

Hemodynamically mediated renal failure

Nonsteroidal anti-inflammatory drugs

Although the widely-used NSAIDs generally are safe and well-tolerated, their nephrotoxic potential is significant in patients in the ICU whose renal blood flow may be compromised by preexisting renal disease, sepsis, heart failure, or other conditions [7]. In situations of decreased renal blood flow, prostaglandin production in the renal cortex and medulla increases to maintain renal afferent arteriolar tone, and thus, antagonizes the renal vasoconstriction that is caused by angiotensin II, norepinephrine, vasopressin, and endothelin [7,8]. Through the inhibition of cyclooxygenase (COX), the enzyme that mediates prostaglandin production from arachidonic acid, NSAIDs decrease the synthesis of the vasodilatory prostaglandins. The ensuing vasoconstriction and renal ischemia result in renal failure [7,9]. Renal effects seem to be dose-, drug-, and duration-related; aspirin is the least likely to cause renal failure, whereas indomethacin is the most likely. Ibuprofen, diclofenac, and naproxen have an intermediate risk for renal dysfunction [9]. The orally and parenterally available ketorolac also may cause ARF and should be used with caution in high-risk patients [7].

The introduction of COX-2–selective NSAIDs was expected to lessen the nephrotoxicity of these agents by preferentially inhibiting the proinflammatory effects of COX-2 and sparing the COX-1 physiologic regulatory mechanisms. Data revealed that COX-2 inhibitors, similar to their nonselective counterparts, also are likely to induce renal failure in high-risk patients [10–13]. COX-2 is expressed constitutively in the kidney and is regulated tightly in response to volume contraction. In a review of the Adverse Event Reporting System, Ahmad and colleagues [10] discovered 122 cases of celecoxib-associated renal failure and 142 cases of rofecoxib-related renal failure. Most patients had risk factors for renal failure (hypertension, diabetes mellitus, congestive heart failure, preexisting renal failure or impairment), which illustrates the fact that COX-2 inhibitors still pose nephrotoxic potential to patients who are at danger for renal dysfunction. COX-2 inhibitors should be used with caution in patients in the ICU because of their underlying risk for renal failure and hemodynamic instability.

Patients who are at risk for NSAID-induced renal failure generally have preexisting renal dysfunction, cardiovascular or severe hepatic disease, compromised renal blood flow, or are taking medications that may potentiate the renal failure (eg, diuretics, aminoglycosides, angiotensin-converting enzyme inhibitors, angiotensin II receptor blockers) [7,9]. In the intensive care setting, NSAID-related ARF usually is hemodynamically mediated, and manifests as a rapid decline in creatinine clearance [7,9]. Renal failure may be seen after only a few dosages, and urine volume and sodium concentration are typically low. NSAIDs also can cause many other renal syndromes, such as nephrotic syndrome, interstitial nephritis, papillary necrosis, and electrolyte and fluid abnormalities [7,9,13]. Usually, renal failure is reversible upon discontinuation of the NSAID and initiation of supportive care measures. If an NSAID must be used in a patient who has poor renal perfusion, a drug with a short half-life that causes less prostaglandin inhibition should be used (eg, aspirin, sulindac) [7].

Vasopressors

Patients in the ICU who are in hypovolemic, septic, or cardiogenic shock are at severe risk for renal failure that is due to poor kidney perfusion. Vasopressor use is common in critically ill patients to support blood pressure and tissue and organ perfusion following volume replacement. The authors' drug use evaluation data revealed that dopamine and epinephrine were among the most commonly used vasopressors in the adult and pediatric ICUs (see Tables 2 and 3). The higher doses of these agents that may be necessary to provide adequate blood pressure support cause vasoconstriction, and thus, may reduce renal blood flow. Prolonged use of vasopressors at elevated doses may result in kidney hypoxia and acute tubular necrosis, mainly in patients who are inadequately fluid resuscitated, because of decreased renal perfusion.

The use of low-dose dopamine (<3 μg/kg/min) has received much attention in critically ill patients. At this dosage, dopamine acts primarily on the dopamine receptors, and results in renal vasculature vasodilation. It was theorized that such vasodilation is helpful in the ARF setting, and studies showed that infusing low-dose dopamine increases glomerular filtration rate and urine output [14–16]; however, this did not improve the outcome in patients who had ARF [17]. The results of major trials in which variable dopamine dosing was used showed that low-dose dopamine (<3 μg/kg/min) did not reduce the need for dialysis or improve overall survival [18,19]. In addition, low-dose dopamine may have detrimental effects, including cardiac dysrhythmias, tissue extravasation, and decreased prolactin production [17,20,21]. Low-dose (so called "renal-dose") dopamine has no role in the management of patients who have existing renal dysfunction. The use of "renal-dose" dopamine is surprisingly common considering the unanimity of evidence that rejects its clinical usefulness. Its use cannot be recommended for "nephroprotection" because the literature does not support this practice.

Tubular nephrotoxicity

Aminoglycosides

The excellent antimicrobial activity of aminoglycosides against gram-negative bacteria explains their continued usage in the management of infections in critically ill patients. The authors' drug use evaluation showed that gentamicin was ordered frequently in their ICUs; its use was more common in pediatric patients. The nephrotoxicity of aminoglycosides has long been recognized and is well documented. The minimally protein–bound aminoglycosides are eliminated primarily by the kidneys through glomerular filtration. These drugs accumulate within renal tubular cortical cells and exert their nephrotoxicity through proximal tubular epithelial cell damage [7,22,23]. The cationic state of the aminoglycosides facilitates their binding to tubular epithelial cells. Intracellular transport results in high concentrations of the aminoglycoside within the lysosomes of the cells [7,22–26]. Cellular functions, such as protein reabsorption, protein synthesis, mitochondrial function, and the sodium-potassium-ATPase pump, are disrupted. In addition to cellular metabolic function interference, aminoglycosides cause cell death when the lysis of lysosomal membranes occurs, which spills lysosomal enzymes, toxins, and the aminoglycoside into the cytosol [22,24].

One of the earliest indicators of proximal tubular damage is enzymuria with brush-border enzymes or other intracellular enzymes [7,23]. Enzymuria is not measured commonly in the clinical setting. Clinical evidence of aminoglycoside nephrotoxicity characteristically manifests within 5 to 10 days after initiation of therapy. Elevations in serum urea nitrogen levels and serum creatinine are seen eventually, and renal failure typically is nonoliguric [7,23]. Usually, renal failure is reversible after cessation of therapy, although normal renal function may take months to return fully.

Potential risk factors for aminoglycoside-associated nephrotoxicity include decreased renal blood flow, volume depletion, age, preexisting renal dysfunction, duration and repeated courses of aminoglycoside therapy, large cumulative doses, and concomitant nephrotoxin administration [7,23,27]. Administering aminoglycosides in higher doses at extended intervals may decrease the nephrotoxicity of these agents. With this dosing strategy, the increased initial drug concentration and prolonged postantibiotic effect allow for a longer dosing interval and a prolonged period of drug-free antibiotic concentration in the serum [23,26]. Limiting aminoglycoside exposure by changing therapy to less toxic antibiotics following organism identification and susceptibility testing also may reduce nephrotoxicity. Aminoglycoside-induced ARF usually is reversible upon early discontinuation of the drug, although renal replacement therapy may be warranted until renal function is restored.

Amphotericin B

Amphotericin B has a broad spectrum of activity, which makes it an attractive option for the treatment of many fungal diseases. Amphotericin B was among the top 100 ordered medications in the authors' neonatal ICU and pediatric cardiothoracic ICU.

The use of amphotericin B is limited by its side effect profile, particularly its nephrotoxicity potential. Renal failure that is induced by amphotericin B is the result of systemic and renal arterial vasoconstriction and subsequent ischemic injury, as well as increased membrane permeability to sodium and potassium that is due to amphotericin binding to and damaging tubular epithelial cells

[24,27–29]. The altered membrane permeability leads to increased oxygen requirements and vasoconstriction results in decreased oxygen delivery to cells. Thus, renal medullary tubular cell necrosis and death occur.

ARF with amphotericin B administration is common; toxic manifestations are elevations in serum urea nitrogen and serum creatinine, along with oliguria. Sodium, potassium, and magnesium wasting also may occur. Risk factors for amphotericin B renal toxicity include preexisting renal insufficiency, concomitant nephrotoxin administration, large individual and cumulative doses, and volume depletion [27,28].

Because patients in the ICU may have several of these risk factors, prevention of amphotericin toxicity is important. Sodium and volume loading help to decrease the nephrotoxicity by reducing vasoconstriction [30]. Avoiding the concurrent administration of other nephrotoxic medications may reduce synergistic nephrotoxicity. Several lipid-based formulations of amphotericin B are available (AmBisome, Abelcet, Amphotec), and may produce less nephrotoxicity than the deoxycholate formulation without affecting clinical effectiveness [31–33]. Although the cost of liposomal products is significantly greater than amphotericin B deoxycholate, their use may be preferred in patients who are at high risk for nephrotoxicity. Several antifungal agents are available that may be alternatives to amphotericin, including fluconazole, itraconazole, voriconazole, and caspofungin.

Radiocontrast dye

Radiocontrast dye usage could not be tracked in the authors' ICU medication use review because of limitations in the ability to collect the data with pharmacy department software; nonetheless, all clinicians recognize the nephrotoxic potential of these agents. Radiocontrast dye causes nephrotoxicity in many ways, including by altering renal hemodynamics and direct damage to renal tubular cells [34]. The presence of preexisting renal disease, diabetes mellitus, hypertension, and advanced age predispose patients to the development of radiocontrast dye nephrotoxicity [35–37]. Patients who are at risk for nephrotoxicity should receive low osmolality contrast dye instead of high osmolality contrast dye because it is less nephrotoxic [38]. Hypovolemia also is associated with the development of radiocontrast dye nephropathy; therefore it is essential to assure adequate hydration before dye administration. It is apparent that the use of sodium chloride infusions alone is superior in the prevention of nephrotoxicity to the coadministration of loop diuretics or mannitol [39]. More recent data suggest that infusion with 154 mEq/L sodium bicarbonate is superior to normal saline infusion (154 mEq/L sodium chloride) in the prevention of radiocontrast dye nephropathy [40]. These data need to be corroborated, but represent a simple preventative therapy that holds great potential. Other therapies to prevent radiocontrast dye nephropathy have been studied, and of these, *N*-acetyl-L-cysteine seems to hold the most promise [41].

The management of TLS involves hydration, correction of metabolic abnormalities, and supportive care for renal failure. Sodium bicarbonate–containing fluids alkalinize the urine and increase the solubility of uric acid by increasing the amount of uric acid in the ionized form. Uric acid is best excreted at a pH of greater than 7 [55]. The xanthine oxidase inhibitor allopurinol prevents the formation of uric acid; dosages of up to 800 mg/d orally have been used. Rasburicase, a recombinant form of urate oxidase, converts already formed uric acid to the more soluble allantoin, and thus, facilitates the excretion of uric acid from the body [54–56]. In some instances, dialysis may be indicated for the treatment of TLS-associated renal failure. Renal replacement therapy should be initiated when preventative measures have been proven inadequate. The goal of dialysis is to correct potassium, calcium, phosphorus, and uric acid abnormalities and to prevent further renal damage [54,55].

Summary

ARF may occur in patients in the ICU because of medications, sepsis, renal hypoperfusion, volume depletion, intrinsic kidney damage, and postrenal obstruction. Although the exact percentage of drug-induced ARF is not known, medications can lead to renal dysfunction by causing acute tubular necrosis, glomerular and tubulointerstitial damage, hemodynamically mediated damage, and obstructive nephropathy. The drug use evaluation that was performed at UMHS showed that known nephrotoxins, such as antimicrobials (aminoglycosides, amphotericin B, penicillins, cephalosporins, acyclovir), and NSAIDs, are used widely in the ICUs. ARF in patients in the ICU is associated with a high risk for mortality. Clinicians must understand that many of the therapeutic agents that are used in the ICU can cause drug-induced renal dysfunction. Early recognition of drug-induced renal dysfunction may alleviate some of the morbidity and mortality that are associated with ARF in the ICU.

Acknowledgments

The authors wish to acknowledge Michael E. McGregory, Strategic Projects Coordinator, University of Michigan Health System, for his assistance in collecting ICU medication usage data.

References

[1] Uchino S, Kellum JA, Bellomo R, et al. Acute renal failure in critically ill patients: a multinational, multicenter study. JAMA 2005;294(7):813–8.
[2] Ympa YP, Sakr Y, Reinhart K, et al. Has mortality from acute renal failure decreased? A systematic review of the literature. Am J Med 2005;118:827–32.

[3] Novis BK, Roizen MF, Aronson S, et al. Association of preoperative risk factors with postoperative acute renal failure. Anesth Analg 1994;78(1):143–9.
[4] Bernieh B, Al Hakim M, Boobes Y, et al. Pattern of acute renal failure in a tertiary hospital in the United Arab Emirates. Transplant Proc 2004;36(6):1780–3.
[5] Micromedex® Healthcare Series. Greenwood Village (CO): Thomson Micromedex (edition expires [3/2006]).
[6] Bhatt-Mehta V, Schumacher RE, Faix RG, et al. Lack of vancomycin-associated nephrotoxicity in newborn infants: a case-control study. Pediatrics 1999;103(4):e48.
[7] Hock R, Anderson RJ. Prevention of drug-induced nephrotoxicity in the intensive care unit. J Crit Care 1995;10(1):33–43.
[8] Perazella MA. Drug-induced renal failure: update on new medications and unique mechanisms of nephrotoxicity. Am J Med 2003;325:349–62.
[9] Whelton A. Nephrotoxicity of nonsteroidal anti-inflammatory drugs: physiologic foundations and clinical implications. Am J Med 1999;106(5B):13S–24S.
[10] Ahmad SR, Kortepeter C, Brinker A, et al. Renal failure associated with the use of celecoxib and rofecoxib. Drug Saf 2002;25(7):537–44.
[11] Morales E, Mucksavage JJ. Cyclooxygenase-2 inhibitor-associated acute renal failure: case report with rofecoxib and review of the literature. Pharmacother 2002;22(10):1317–21.
[12] Perazella MA, Tray K. Selective cyclooxygenase-2 inhibitors: a pattern of nephrotoxicity similar to traditional nonsteroidal anti-inflammatory drugs. Am J Med 2001;111:64–7.
[13] Gambaro G, Perazella MA. Adverse renal effects of anti-inflammatory agents: evaluation of selective and nonselective cyclooxygenase inhibitors. J Int Med 2003;253:643–52.
[14] Harper L, Savage COS. The use of dopamine in acute renal failure. Clin Nephrol 1997;47: 347–9.
[15] Richer M, Robert S, Lebel M. Renal hemodynamics during norepinephrine and low-dose dopamine infusion in man. Crit Care Med 1996;24:1150–6.
[16] Schaer GL, Fink MP, Parrillo JE. Norepinephrine alone versus norepinephrine plus low-dose dopamine: enhanced renal blood flow with combination vasopressor therapy. Crit Care Med 1985;13:492–6.
[17] Power DA, Duggan J, Brady HR. Renal-dose (low-dose) dopamine for the treatment of sepsis-related and other forms of acute renal failure: ineffective and probably dangerous. Clin Exp Pharmacol Physiol Suppl 1999;26:S23–8.
[18] Chertow GM, Sayegh MH, Allgren RL, et al. Is the administration of dopamine associated with adverse or favorable outcomes in acute renal failure? Am J Med 1996;101:49–53.
[19] Marik PE, Iglesias J. Low-dose dopamine does not prevent acute renal failure in patients with septic shock and oliguria. NORASEPT II Study Investigators. Am J Med 1999;107: 387–90.
[20] Argalious M, Motta P, Khandwala F, et al. "Renal dose" dopamine is associated with the risk of new-onset atrial fibrillation after cardiac surgery. Crit Care Med 2005;33(6):1327–32.
[21] Bailey AR, Burchett KR. Effect of low-dose dopamine on serum concentrations of prolactin in critically ill patients. Br J Anaesth 1997;78:97–9.
[22] Mingeot-Leclercq MP, Tulkens PM. Aminoglycosides: nephrotoxicity. Antimicrob Agents Chemother 1999;43(5):1003–12.
[23] Swan SK. Aminoglycoside nephrotoxicity. Semin Nephrol 1997;17:27–33.
[24] Fanos V, Cataldi L. Renal transport of antibiotics and nephrotoxicity: a review. J Chemother 2001;13(5):461–72.
[25] Nagai J, Takan M. Molecular aspects of renal handling of aminoglycosides and strategies for preventing the nephrotoxicity. Drug Metab Pharmacokinet 2004;19(3):159–70.
[26] Olsen KM, Rudis MI, Rebuck JA, et al. Effect of once-daily dosing vs. multiple daily dosing of tobramycin on enzyme markers of nephrotoxicity. Crit Care Med 2004;32(8):1678–82.
[27] Joannidis M. Drug-induced renal failure in the ICU. Int J Artif Org 2004;27(12):1034–42.
[28] Deray G. Amphotericin B nephrotoxicity. J Antimicrob Chemother 2002;49(Suppl S1):37–41.
[29] Tiphine M, Letscher-Bru V, Herbrecht R. Amphotericin B and its new formulations:

pharmacologic characteristics, clinical efficacy, and tolerability. Transpl Infect Dis 1999;1: 273–83.
[30] Anderson CM. Sodium chloride treatment of amphotericin B nephrotoxicity—standard of care? West J Med 1995;162(4):313–7.
[31] Sharkey PK, Graybill JR, Johnson ES, et al. Amphotericin B lipid complex compared with amphotericin B in the treatment of cryptococcal meningitis in patients with AIDS. Clin Infect Dis 1996;22(2):315–21.
[32] Walsh TJ, Finberg RW, Arndt C, et al. Liposomal amphotericin B for empirical therapy in patients with persistent fever and neutropenia. N Engl J Med 1999;340(10):764–71.
[33] White MH, Bowden RA, Sandler RA, et al. Randomized, double-blind clinical trial of amphotericin B colloidal dispersion vs. amphotericin B in the empirical treatment of fever and neutropenia. Clin Infect Dis 1998;27(2):296–302.
[34] Goldenberg I, Matetzky S. Nephropathy induced by contrast media: pathogenesis, risk factors and preventative strategies. CMAJ 2005;172(11):1461–71.
[35] Iakovou I, Dangas G, Mehran R, et al. Impact of gender on the incidence and outcome of contrast-induced nephropathy after percutaneous coronary intervention. J Invasive Cardiol 2003; 15(1):18–22.
[36] McCullough PA, Wolyn R, Rocher LL, et al. Acute renal failure after coronary intervention: incidence, risk factors, and relationship to mortality. Am J Med 1997;103(5):368–75.
[37] Rihal CS, Textor SC, Grill DE, et al. Incidence and prognostic importance of acute renal failure after percutaneous coronary intervention. Circulation 2002;105(19):2259–64.
[38] Barrett BJ, Carlisle EJ. Metaanalysis of the relative nephrotoxicity of high- and low-osmolality iodinated contrast media. Radiology 1993;188(1):171–8.
[39] Stevens MA, McCullough PA, Tobin KJ, et al. A prospective randomized trial of prevention measures in patients at high risk for contrast nephropathy: results of the P.R.I.N.C.E Study. Prevention of Radiocontrast Induced Nephropathy Clinical Evaluation. J Am Coll Cardiol 1999; 33(2):403–11.
[40] Merten GJ, Burgess WP, Gray LV, et al. Prevention of contrast-induced nephropathy with sodium bicarbonate: a randomized controlled trial. JAMA 2004;291(19):2328–34.
[41] Goldenberg I, Schechter M, Matetzky S, et al. Oral acetylcysteine as an adjunct to saline hydration for the prevention of contrast-induced nephropathy following coronary angiography. A randomized controlled trial and review of the current literature. Eur Heart J 2004;25(3): 212–8.
[42] Markowitz GS, Perazella MA. Drug-induced renal failure: a focus on tubulointerstitial disease. Clin Chim Acta 2005;351:31–47.
[43] Michel DM, Kelly CJ. Acute interstitial nephritis. J Am Soc Nephrol 1998;9(3):506–15.
[44] Sakarcan A, Marcille R, Stallworth J. Antibiotic-induced recurring interstitial nephritis. Pediatr Nephrol 2002;17:50–1.
[45] Toto RD. Review: acute tubulointerstitial nephritis. Am J Med Sci 1999;299(6):392–410.
[46] Pill MW, O'Neill CV, Chapman MM, et al. Suspected acute interstitial nephritis induced by piperacillin-tazobactam. Pharmacother 1997;17(1):166–9.
[47] Izzedine H, Launay-Vacher V, Deray G. Antiviral drug-induced nephrotoxicity. Am J Kidney Dis 2005;45(5):804–17.
[48] Perazella MA. Crystal-induced acute renal failure. Am J Med 1999;106:459–65.
[49] Bean B, Aeppli D. Adverse effects of high-dose intravenous acyclovir in ambulatory patients with acute herpes zoster. J Infect Dis 1985;151(2):362–5.
[50] Brigden D, Rosling AE, Woods NC. Renal function after acyclovir intravenous injection. Am J Med 1982;73:182–5.
[51] Keeney RE, Kirk LE, Bridgen D. Acyclovir tolerance in humans. Am J Med 1982;73:176–81.
[52] Krasny HC, Liao SH, deMiranda P, et al. Influence of hemodialysis on acyclovir pharmacokinetics in patients with chronic renal failure. Am J Med 1982;73(1A):202–4.
[53] Laskin OL, Longstreth JA, Whelton A, et al. Effect of renal failure on the pharmacokinetics of acyclovir. Am J Med 1982;73(1A):197–201.

[54] Cairo MS, Bishop M. Tumour lysis syndrome: new therapeutic strategies and classification. Br J Haematol 2004;127:3–11.

[55] Davidson MB, Thakkar S, Hix JK, et al. Pathophysiology, clinical consequences, and treatment of tumor lysis syndrome. Am J Med 2005;116:546–64.

[56] Lameire NH, Flombaum CS, Moreau D, et al. Acute renal failure in cancer patients. Ann Med 2005;37:13–25.

ELSEVIER
SAUNDERS

Crit Care Clin 22 (2006) 375–381

CRITICAL
CARE
CLINICS

Index

Note: Page numbers of article titles are in **boldface** type.

A

0749-0704/06/$ – see front matter
doi:10.1016/S0749-0704(06)00039-X

Changing Your Address?

Make sure your subscription changes too! When you notify us of your new address, you can help make our job easier by including an exact copy of your Clinics label number with your old address (see illustration below.) This number identifies you to our computer system and will speed the processing of your address change. Please be sure this label number accompanies your old address and your corrected address—you can send an old Clinics label with your number on it or just copy it exactly and send it to the address listed below.

We appreciate your help in our attempt to give you continuous coverage. Thank you.

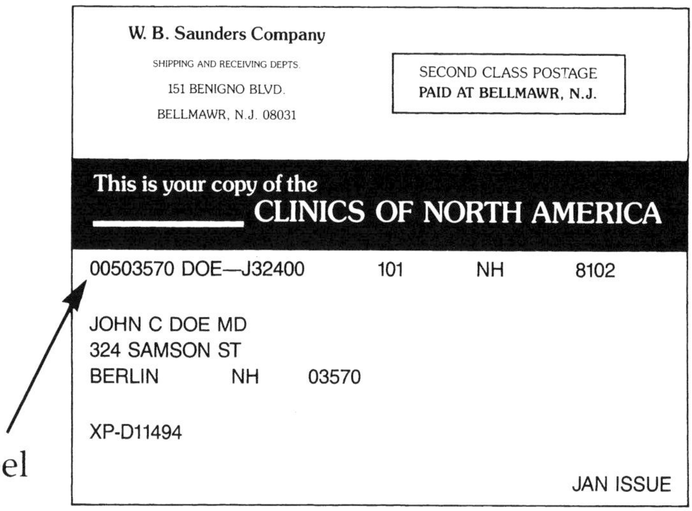

Your Clinics Label Number

Copy it exactly or send your label along with your address to:

W.B. Saunders Company, Customer Service
Orlando, FL 32887-4800
Call Toll Free 1-800-654-2452

Please allow four to six weeks for delivery of new subscriptions and for processing address changes.